Undoing Motherhood

Families in Focus

For a list of all the titles in the series, please see the
last page of the book.

Undoing Motherhood

Collaborative Reproduction and the Deinstitutionalization of U.S. Maternity

KATHERINE M. JOHNSON

Rutgers University Press
New Brunswick, Camden, and Newark, New Jersey
London and Oxford

Library of Congress Cataloging-in-Publication Data
Names: Johnson, Katherine M. (Sociologist), author.
Title: Undoing motherhood : collaborative reproduction and the
deinstitutionalization of US maternity / Katherine M. Johnson.
Description: New Brunswick, New Jersey : Rutgers University Press, [2023] |
Series: Families in focus series | Includes bibliographical references and index.
Identifiers: LCCN 2022028688 | ISBN 9781978808676 (paperback ; alk. paper) |
ISBN 9781978808683 (cloth ; alk. paper) | ISBN 9781978808690 (epub) |
ISBN 9781978808713 (pdf)
Subjects: LCSH: Motherhood—United States. | Human reproductive technology—
Social aspects—United States. | Reproductive rights—United States.
Classification: LCC HQ 759 .J635 2023 | DDC 306.874/30973—dc23/eng/20220727
LC record available at https://lccn.loc.gov/2022028688

A British Cataloging-in-Publication record for this book is available
from the British Library.

References to internet websites (URLs) were accurate at the time of writing. Neither
the author nor Rutgers University Press is responsible for URLs that may have
expired or changed since the manuscript was prepared.

rutgersuniversitypress.org

For my family

Contents

Undoing Motherhood

1

A New Maternity Uncertainty?

In 2012, I gave birth to my first child. My spouse and I had conceived naturally—that is, if "naturally" includes careful planning and surveillance of the best time to have a baby, both in terms of life course timing and menstrual cycle tracking. My labor began, rather serendipitously, at 11:00 P.M. on my due date. Everything went largely according to plan. I delivered at a local hospital with minimal interventions, as requested in our birth plan. I began nursing my baby while her cord was still uncut, waiting for my placenta to emerge. My spouse and doula were both by my side. We were all relieved, exhausted, and elated after my eighteen hours of labor. When I think back, I realize that my biggest fear going into labor was that I would not know which baby was mine once she came out of my body. I found myself wondering if I was already a bad mother because I had little faith in my ability to pick out my infant from other babies in the hospital nursery. Would some sort of maternal instinct kick in, allowing me to recognize her once she was outside my body?

I recall examining her from head to toe after she was born, memorizing her face, her hair, her eyes. I was relieved by the hospital protocol of immediately putting an identification and security band on her ankle, linked to my own patient wristband. It also helped that on her first trip out of my sight after birth, her father carried her so carefully in his arms. He also stayed at the nursery, watching while she was weighed, bathed, and charted, before she was returned to my side in a clear bassinet. The next day, we filled out paperwork to order her birth certificate. My maternity was taken for granted. She came from my body. My spouse was automatically listed as her father because we were married, and he voluntarily declared his paternity on the hospital forms. His bio-genetic paternity was also never in question, especially after the baby came out of me with a full head of the darkest brown, nearly black, curls—looking just like him. Her birth certificate came in the mail several weeks later. Our family unit was firmly established. Our story is the typical story of integrated biosocial reproduction. The rest of this book, however, is the story of what happens when this order of things becomes disrupted by technological interventions—interventions that move reproduction outside and between different bodies. My own fear of potentially not knowing which baby was mine once she left my body is a very real fear that becomes extended and amplified in collaborative forms of reproduction in the post–in vitro fertilization (IVF) era.

In July 1978, the first so-called test-tube baby was born from IVF, under the careful supervision of Drs. Edwards and Steptoe in the United Kingdom. Three years later, Drs. Howard and Georgianna Jones successfully repeated this feat in the United States: Elizabeth Jordan Carr was born in 1981, in Norfolk, Virginia. These early IVF babies are now approaching middle age. The decades since their births have been filled with other innovations in reproductive medicine, such as egg donation, embryo donation, gestational surrogacy, intracytoplasmic sperm injection (ICSI), uterine implants, mitochondrial replacement—the list goes on. IVF created a paradigm shift for infertility treatment and assisted reproduction. The medical and scientific ability to extract, fertilize, and store reproductive cells outside the human body opened up a new set of opportunities for family building—especially for people with medical or social barriers to reproduction such as biomedical infertility or lack of a reproductive partner.[1] But this newfound mobility of gametes and embryos has also prompted conflicts about responsibility for, rights to, and control over, reproductive cells.

One major arena where such conflicts play out is that of parentage rights. The United States provides a distinct national context for addressing both parentage and collaborative reproduction. Compared to other nations, it has a relatively laissez-faire approach to regulating what has unfolded as a largely privatized fertility industry (Markens 2007; L. Martin 2009 and 2015). Any sort of regulatory approaches to parentage are also decentralized because family law is the purview of the states (Cahn 2013; Crockin and Jones 2010; Heidt-Forsythe 2018). Furthermore, while most U.S. states have passed statutes that clarify paternity in sperm donation, there is significantly less legal clarification of maternity in egg donation, embryo donation, and gestational surrogacy (Nejaime 2017)—the three techniques I explore in this book. These all fall under the umbrella of 'collaborative' or 'third-party' reproduction, which refer to reproductive assistance from an outside party (such as a gamete or embryo donor or gestational surrogate) who does not intend to be a legal or social parent to the resulting child. Throughout this book, I opt to use the term 'collaborative reproduction' rather than 'third-party reproduction.' The latter is implicitly heteronormative, emerging from the notion that the third party is in addition to a husband and wife in an infertile couple. By contrast, collaborative reproduction captures what is essential to the process (i.e., the involvement of additional parties) but is also more inclusive of various family forms being created.

Egg donation involves retrieving oocytes from a healthy young donor, followed by in vitro fertilization with sperm from the recipient's partner or a donor, and then transferring the resulting embryo or embryos into the recipient's uterus for gestation (American Society for Reproductive Medicine [ASRM] 2012). The egg donor is genetically linked to the child, but the recipient woman typically carries the pregnancy and gives birth. Embryo donation transfers a fully created embryo to the recipient's uterus, with the embryo often donated by a heterosexual couple who have already gone through infertility treatment and have excess embryos (ASRM 2012). In embryo donation, similar to egg donation, the recipient woman usually carries the pregnancy and gives birth. Finally, there are two types of surrogacy arrangements: traditional surrogacy, in which the surrogate provides both the egg and carries the pregnancy, and gestational surrogacy, in which the surrogate carries the pregnancy but has no genetic connection to the child (ASRM 2012). In gestational surrogacy, the intended social mother (the woman who intends to raise the child) may provide an egg, or a donated egg or embryo may be used. In my analysis, I focus on gestational surrogacy, which is now more common than traditional surrogacy. This shift is due to the technological developments that allowed for an embryo to be transferred into another woman's body, as well as to the fact that gestational surrogacy makes many intended parents feel more legally and socially secure in their parentage because it disrupts the genetic tie between surrogate and child (Jacobson 2016; Ragone 1999).

These collaborative reproduction techniques can produce four possible maternal-child connections: genetic, via eggs; gestational, through pregnancy; social and psychological, through parenting or intent to parent; and legal, through established rights and responsibilities. Typically, these connections are all with one person, with adoption being a common exception. However, in adoption, there is not usually a question about the maternity of the woman giving birth: she maintains the status of birth mother, even while relinquishing the status of legal and social mother. Whether this maternal status is kept a secret or not is historically and culturally contingent, as is whether the woman giving birth is encouraged to forget about her birth maternity and move on (Fessler 2006; Solinger 1994). In collaborative reproduction, however, multiple women may variously contribute to conception, gestation, and birth, and then legal and social responsibilities for rearing the child. What does this multiplicity of contributions mean for conceptualizing maternity?

First, systematically privileging any specific connection undermines the legitimacy of other connections. For example, some people argue for using paternity as an analogy to solve the problem: the combination of man, sperm, and paternity suggests the equivalent combination of woman, egg, and maternity. But what are the implications of viewing genetic ties between a woman and child as the best way to establish maternity? Doing this would undermine gestational or purely social forms of maternity in which mothers have partial or no biological connection to their child. Second, with such an array of possible connections, should there only be one 'true' mother of a child? These are big questions, and clearly I am not the first person to grapple with them. Yet feminist scholars and family sociologists have rarely made the implications of collaborative reproduction for maternity the central problem of their analysis.[2]

My goal in this book is not to provide some sort of definitive answer about what constitutes maternity. Spoiler: there is no epiphany in these pages about how to best decide who is the mom or how to reveal the essence of maternity. Instead, my purpose is to shine a light on maternity as part of the institution of motherhood—a part that often gets overlooked even with the proliferation of scholarship on motherhood in the past several decades (Arendell 2000; Glenn, Chang, and Forcey 1994; Hays 1996; Jeremiah 2006; Kawash 2011). I use collaborative reproduction as a lens (or maybe a flashlight) to peer into the dark corners of how our culture thinks about maternity and what happens when we disrupt its taken-for-granted biological roots.

Research Questions and Guiding Frameworks

In my analysis, I focus on the distinct but overlapping social worlds of law and reproductive medicine. These two worlds are intimately involved with collaborative reproduction as they assist people on their family-building journeys. These worlds also have to grapple with the implications of postmodern family building. Here are my driving questions throughout this book:

1. How has collaborative reproduction affected maternity definitions and designation, both formally and informally?
2. Given the newer, diverse paths to maternity, who gets to be legally and socially recognized as an authentic mother to a given child?
3. Are some maternal connections considered more legally or socially authentic than others?

One of my major arguments, which serves as a touchstone throughout, is that collaborative reproduction introduces a new type of maternity uncertainty.[3] By this I mean that there is increasing cultural uncertainty about what does and should constitute maternity. Defining maternity is an important issue because it sets the foundation for legal and social rights and responsibilities in a parent-child relationship. Definitions also clearly mark boundaries between family and nonfamily. The issue of maternity uncertainty is connected to, but also quite different from, the long-standing cultural trope of uncertain paternity (Milanich 2017) or paternity nonconfidence (K. Anderson 2006). There is a difference between not knowing who the progenitor of a specific child is versus not having a concise social and legal guide for how to delegate the role of parent to someone. My concern is with the latter. More than two decades ago, Sarah Franklin (1995, 335) characterized assisted reproduction as "postmodern procreation," arguing that these technologies ushered in a "crisis of legitimacy . . . in traditional beliefs about parenthood, procreation, and kinship." In this book, I show how traditional biolegal maternity, often viewed as an irrefutable, bedrock relationship, is undergoing a particular cultural crisis because we lack consistent "social and legal rules" (Milanich 2017, 25) to guide emerging scenarios in collaborative reproduction.

The sociologist Andrew Cherlin (1978 and 2004) used the concept of deinstitutionalization to describe broad changes in the American family in the late twentieth and early twenty-first centuries, including those related to divorce, remarriage, stepparenting, and cohabitation and the increasing social separation between marriage and childbearing. He argued that there was a "weakening of social norms . . . that define . . . behavior in a social institution" (2004, 848). Cherlin also pointed to the emergence of new family situations for which people lacked consistent norms and institutional support, defining these situations as "incomplete institutions" (1978). More recently, the sociologists Rosanna Hertz and Margaret Nelson (2019) used the framework of deinstitutionalization to examine new family-like relationships emerging when individuals from multiple families find out that they had the same sperm donor. I borrow and build on these ideas to look at maternity as one piece of kinship and family. In the post-IVF era, traditional biolegal maternity is undergoing a sort of deinstitutionalization, being replaced by a newer, incomplete institution. The newness and incompleteness offer more possibilities for maternal-child relationships, but not necessarily the same protections as maternity's traditional form.

Scholars working on the relationships among science, law, and technology have frequently pointed to the issue of 'cultural lag.' Reproductive medicine has made numerous scientific and technological leaps, and the law and social norms might simply need to catch up. In his classic sociological work, William Ogburn (1922, 197) defined cultural lag as the gap between the introduction of new material conditions (e.g., technological innovations) and cultural adjustment. The gap is a time of sense making and "maladjustment," when older cultural norms are still in use but do not fit with changing social conditions. People must make meaning and order out of new circumstances that have disrupted the taken-for-granted flow of activities (Blumer 1969; Lauer and Handel 1977). As Karl Weick (1995, 14–15) observes, "to engage in sensemaking is to construct, filter, frame, create facticity. . . . [Sensemaking approaches] reality as an ongoing accomplishment that takes form when people make retrospective sense of situations in which they find themselves and their creations."

One approach to the cultural lag between law and reproductive medicine is to speed up legal change to create a better fit with changing family conditions. Another, more realistic, view is that there is not simply a neutral lag time before laws inevitably catch up, but a tug-of-war between different ideologies of the family: a traditional ideology in which the family is conceived of as a social whole that is hierarchical, fixed, and based in biogenetic and heterosexual relations, versus a modern family ideology that favors egalitarianism, individualism, and choice (Cahn and Carbone 2010; Dolgin 1997; Weston 1991). One issue that came to light in my research for this book is that most physicians who initially conducted procedures like artificial insemination with donor sperm

(AID) and IVF were not intentionally trying to create new family forms or revolutionize cultural definitions about families. Rather, many were aiming to do quite the opposite and acted to conceal any such medically assisted deviations from the traditional, bio-genetic family.

Technological Trajectories in Assisted and Collaborative Reproduction

One major point that I focus on in my analysis is that maternity and paternity have been transformed in different ways by assisted and collaborative reproduction (Figure 1.1). Traditionally, men are assumed to largely experience reproduction as a disconnected, disembodied process (Rothman 1989; Almeling and Waggoner 2013). Aside from sexual activity, men are physically and symbolically distanced from conception and gestation. As expectant fathers, men were also historically excluded from participating in childbirth (Dye 1980). For women, reproduction is viewed as more connected and embodied: women's bodies are intimately involved throughout pregnancy and during the postpartum period, through breast-feeding and recovering physically and mentally from childbirth. Describing the gendered experience of pregnancy, the sociologist Barbara Katz Rothman (1989, 98) observed: "women's experience of this growth from a cell to a person is continuous; men's experience is discontinuous—in goes a seed, out comes a baby."

Early treatments for infertility did not change this gendered relationship to reproduction. These treatments relied mostly on hormonal and drug therapies, surgical therapies to correct blocked or otherwise inadequate functioning of the reproductive organs, or artificial insemination using the husband's sperm (Barnes 2014; Research Correlating Committee of the American Society for the Study of Sterility 1951). However, these therapies simply did not work in certain cases—such as those involving severe male factor infertility, in which men did not make any (viable) sperm; gamete incompatibility that might increase the couple's risk of

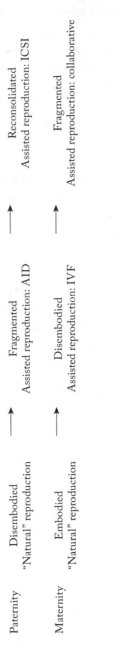

FIG. 1.1. Technological trajectories for paternity and maternity

Paternity	Disembodied "Natural" reproduction	Fragmented Assisted reproduction: AID	→ Reconsolidated Assisted reproduction: ICSI
Maternity	Embodied "Natural" reproduction	Disembodied Assisted reproduction: IVF	→ Fragmented Assisted reproduction: collaborative

transmitting a genetic disorder; or Rh factor discordance between partners that might make pregnancy and birth dangerous to the pregnant woman, fetus, or both (Research Correlating Committee of the American Society for the Study of Sterility 1951). When physicians began to use donor insemination as a new therapy, they created a new phase for men's reproductive role: fragmentation. The technique of AID created a form of intentional "split paternity" (Guttmacher, Haman, and MacLeod 1950, 264) between the socio-legal and the biological paternal role.

During the 1970s and 1980s, the main users of AID began shifting away from heterosexual, infertile couples, as lesbian and single women increasingly sought out family-building options (Spar 2006; Agigian 2004). During this same period, reproductive medicine developed many ways to extract and micromanipulate sperm from male infertility patients (Barnes 2014). These techniques offered the possibility of genetic paternity even in more intractable cases of male infertility. Andrea Laws-King and colleagues from the Monash Medical Center in Australia (1987) reported the first successful fertilization experiment involving microinjection of single spermatozoon beneath the zona pellucida of mature oocytes. By 1992, this method, known as ICSI, was regularly practiced in reproductive medicine (Practice Committee of the American Society for Reproductive Medicine and Society for Assisted Reproductive Technology 2012). ICSI revolutionized the treatment of male infertility. All it took was a single "good" sperm. Men with reduced sperm motility or abnormal sperm morphology could now hope to fertilize an egg with this extra assistance (Laws-King et al. 1987). As Drs. Kamischke and Nieschlag noted (1999, 1): "for patients long considered untreatable, a chance of paternity has become reality." Even men with complete absence of sperm in their ejaculate could have a chance. By the early 2000s, practitioners had at least six different techniques available for retrieving sperm from various parts of men's reproductive systems (Schlegel 2004; Lebovic, Gordon, and Taylor 2014). ICSI prompted a renewed emphasis on the reconsolidation of biological and sociolegal paternity for male infertility patients. As an indication of its medical and cultural

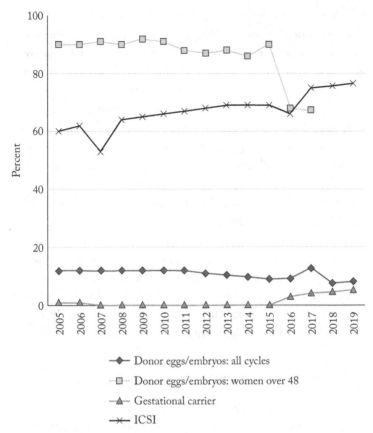

FIG. 1.2. Percent of IVF cycles using ICSI techniques, 2005–2019

Legend for figure:
- Donor eggs/embryos: all cycles
- Donor eggs/embryos: women over 48
- Gestational carrier
- ICSI

significance, national summary data on IVF clinics show that physicians consistently used ICSI techniques with over half of all IVF cycles (53–69 percent) between 2005 and 2016 (Centers for Disease Control and Prevention [CDC], ASRM, and Society for Assisted Reproductive Technology [SART], 2007–2018) (Figure 1.2).

In contrast to women's typically connected and embodied relationship to reproduction, new developments in reproductive medicine began disembodying parts of the process. The successful introduction of IVF in the late 1970s moved fertilization and pre-embryo development from the inner confines of women's bodies to the medical laboratory. Later techniques built on this foundation to move other elements of the reproductive process outside, and between, women's bodies through collaborative reproduction. The first egg donation pregnancy and subsequent live birth followed in 1984 in Australia (Lutjen et al. 1984), and the first successful gestational surrogacy pregnancy took place in 1985 in the United States (Utian et al. 1985). These techniques created not only partial or full reproductive disembodiment, but also the fragmentation of maternity into genetic, gestational, social, and legal components. Although use of collaborative reproduction is relatively lower than that of IVF-only cycles, national summary data show that donor eggs are consistently used in 12–13 percent of all IVF procedures (Figure 1.2). For women older than forty-eight, donor eggs are used in more than 90 percent of IVF cycles (CDC, ASRM, and SART, 2007–2018). IVF patients are least likely to use gestational surrogacy of all the collaborative options. The same national summary data show that at most, 3 percent of IVF cycles involve a gestational carrier, but this number is more typically below 1 percent of all IVF cycles annually.

Legal Responses to Collaborative Reproduction

The connections between technological and legal aspects of collaborative reproduction are complex. As I discuss in greater detail in chapter 3, there were many initial conflicts between AI and legal paternity, particularly when using donor sperm. However, within a few decades, these conflicts seemed to fade into the background, becoming largely resolved—at least for heterosexual married couples. Yet there are continuing cultural and legal conflicts over collaborative reproduction and maternity. Why do these differences exist? For one thing, AID has been around for much longer: its first use was credited to the American physician William Pancoast in the late 1800s (Arny and Quagliarello 1987). But time is only one dimension of understanding cultural reception to new technologies. Another perspective here is that the legal framework in place to establish paternity for the child of a married woman—known as the marital *presumption of paternity*—was quite compatible with AID. Physicians simply had to follow some rules to ensure this compatibility, including the husband's consent to the procedure, physician supervision, strict anonymity among all parties, and nondisclosure to the donor-conceived child, extended family, and community. Thus, paternity as a legal concept was already quite flexible and adaptable, intended to shore up biological uncertainty with legal certainty (Singer 2006). The biological facts of conception did not have to match the legal facts of parentage. The conflict between collaborative reproduction and legal maternity is not so easily resolved. Collaborative reproduction threatens to destabilize maternity precisely because traditionally maternity has been defined more narrowly and rigidly, relying on the *presumption of biology*. Under this presumption, a woman who gives birth is the legal mother of the child: law and biology are united. This traditional framework leads to maternity uncertainty when we unmoor maternity from biology, partially or wholly, and try to alter or expand the range of possible conditions for establishing a maternal-child relationship.

AID AND THE MARITAL PRESUMPTION OF PATERNITY

Establishing paternity is an enduring social and legal problem. Ways to assess biological paternity through blood testing were first available in the 1930s to rule out men whose blood types did not match that of the child. DNA testing, as a way to rule in possible fathers, was available by the late twentieth century (Rudavsky 1999). Before paternity testing became available, paternity certainty relied on strict control over women's sexual behavior, including women's virginity at the time of marriage and complete sexual fidelity during marriage (Engels 2001; Rothman 1989). If these conditions could be met, then any pregnancy the woman had during the marriage could certainly be attributed to her husband. Notably this did not require men's premarital abstinence or sexual fidelity during marriage—a double standard that is an inherent part of patriarchal kinship systems (Rothman 1989). One problem remained: without the ability to control women's bodies and behaviors absolutely, there was still a degree of uncertainty about biological paternity. American courts and legislatures resolved this remaining uncertainty by borrowing the British legal practice of the marital presumption of paternity. Any children born to a woman during her marriage were considered legitimate children of her husband. British common law practice had sought to "carefully [guard] against bastardizing children" (Rudavsky 1999, 127) who had been born to married women. The British tradition emanated from two legal rules, which held that a child was legitimate if a married woman became pregnant while her husband was anywhere within the British Empire (the Lord Hargreave Rule, also known as the Seven Seas Rule), and that spouses could not testify in court about not having access to one another during the period of the child's conception (the Lord Mansfield Rule). Both rules operated in Britain for centuries to inform legal paternity. For instance, the latter rule was thought to have "originated in Roman doctrine," although it was not formally codified in British law until the eighteenth century (Rudavsky 1999, 127).

American law was decidedly influenced by this British tradition and developed its own variant of the marital presumption of paternity, aiming to shore up the nuclear family and protect the welfare of children (Singer 2006). The issue of child welfare was crucial because a child who had been declared illegitimate was treated both legally and socially as a second-class citizen in the United States. Technically, the illegitimate child became "'fillius nullus' . . . the 'son of nobody' . . . no longer entitled to support or inheritance from either parent" (Singer 2006, 249). More frequently, however, this translated into men not having to legally recognize or support their illegitimate children or bestow an inheritance on them, and the social ostracization of both mothers and children (Brumberg 1984). The marital presumption created a precedent for understanding paternity as a conceptual relationship: paternity referenced biology, implied by the sexual marital relationship, but it was not ultimately reduced to biology (Singer 2006). The only way to disprove paternity under the American marital presumption was to show evidence that the husband was "absent, impotent, or sterile" (Kaebnick 2004, 49) during the purported time of conception.

Many U.S. physicians saw donor insemination as a therapeutic option for infertile, married couples to have wanted children. But using donor sperm was also direct evidence that the husband was not the biological father of the resulting child. How could physicians treat male infertility without openly disrupting the marital presumption? During the early twentieth century, medical practitioners and professionals in other fields such as law and psychology expressed numerous concerns about how AID threatened to undermine the institutions of marriage and family. Despite these initial anxieties, by the mid-1990s more than two-thirds of the states had enacted statutes addressing paternity via donor insemination (Seibel and Crockin 1996). At the time of this writing, more than three-fourths of the states, as well as the District of Columbia, have statutes addressing paternity and AID (Nejaime 2017). Most statutes recognize men as the legal fathers of their AID-conceived children if they are married to the recipient woman (i.e., the woman being inseminated) and consent to the procedure, and if a licensed physician performs it. AID, then, is quite compatible with the marital presumption of paternity: both define paternity based on the man's relationship to the mother of the child, not biological paternity itself. One aspect in which AID challenged the traditional presumption of paternity was the explicit evidence (i.e., donor sperm), which directly refuted the presumption of a biological relationship between father and child. The work-around here was the mutual agreement to expand the notion of legitimate paternity to include AID, requiring the husband's consent, physician supervision, and ultimately the blessing of the state. Once codified into law, and with great emphasis on anonymity and secrecy, this expansion of paternity did not pose much threat to the traditional biogenetic family.

COLLABORATIVE REPRODUCTION AND THE BIOLOGICAL PRESUMPTION OF MATERNITY

In contrast to the more conceptual presumption of paternity, giving birth has historically been the main proof of a maternal-child relationship (Kindregan 2009; Stumpf 1986). This *presumption of biology* is rooted in the notion that pregnancy and birth are empirically observable and therefore considered to be irrefutable facts of maternity. The legal scholar Andrea Stumpf noted that maternity has not often caused the same degree of controversy as paternity: "the mother's identity was clear as long as the birth itself was observed" (1986, 187).[4] Biological maternity has therefore been more centrally and rigidly codified for bestowing legal maternity. This codification is exemplified by the legal concept of *mater semper certa*, which dates from Roman times and can be translated as "the mother is always certain" (D'Alton-Harrison 2014, 357; see also Berend and Guerzoni 2021). Yet because women make multiple biological contributions via both genetics and gestation, in the post-IVF era maternity can be fragmented into even more pieces than paternity through assisted and collaborative reproduction. In light of this, how should maternity be legally and socially conceptualized?

One possibility is to define maternity as the genetic relationship between a mother and child. Proponents of this approach aim to make maternity basically equivalent to paternity through the genetic contribution to reproduction. Critics of this approach argue that defining parentage through genetics is reductionist: it overlooks the psychosocial bond and creates a false equivalency between paternity and maternity, ignoring the fact that women's bodies are more involved than men's in reproduction (L. Anderson 2009; Rothman 1989). Simply providing an egg does not necessarily make someone a mother. Others have argued for an emphasis on the gestational relationship, establishing pregnancy as a major element of maternity and countering the genetic approach. For example, Rothman has argued that we should not simply reduce women's reproductive contribution to "the seed" (i.e., gamete) that men have traditionally claimed through patriarchal ideologies. She notes that the "seed" theory also reflects ownership or control over genetic material and, by extension, children. Motherhood has never been about ownership, nor should we want any parent-child relationship to be. Rothman's emphasis on gestation is not intended to reduce maternity to another form of biological connection. She views gestation as both a metaphor for, and a tangible instance of, maternal nurturance and care. One variation on the gestational approach is the legal scholar Leslie Bender's (2006) labor-based, relational, child-centered standard of maternity. In this view, the woman who contributes the greatest labor in creating the child should have priority in being recognized as the legal mother. If she has a partner, they are also awarded parentage indirectly through her maternal status. This approach privileges pregnancy as the greatest amount of labor contributing to the creation and development of a child. It also recognizes pregnancy as the initial, enduring bond. Subsequently, according to Bender, the best way to promote stability for the child is to continue that preexisting bond after birth with legal parentage.

Stepping beyond the genetic-gestational divide, others have argued for parental intent as a precursor to any embodied or biological involvement (L. Anderson 2009; Dolgin 2000; Stumpf 1986). Stumpf (1986) argued for using procreative intent to determine maternity in collaborative reproduction, based on a stage theory of procreative rights where there are discrete moments (stages) throughout the reproductive process. In this view, procreative intent is the ultimate originator of the collaborative reproductive process, providing the crucial foundation for bringing a child into being. Without intent, the parties presumably would not have come together to begin with, and the child would not exist. Stumpf also argued that intent provides evidence of acting in the child's best interest: someone highly motivated to have a child should theoretically be highly motivated to care about that child's well-being. Notably, Stumpf's argument (and others in this vein) is meant specifically to apply to collaborative reproduction, not to reproduction in general. When 45 percent of U.S. pregnancies are unintended (Finer and Zolna 2016), it is hard to make the case that intention is foundational to all reproduction.

The concept of intent has become discursively institutionalized in the U.S. fertility industry with the language of intended parents, a term often used in gestational surrogacy arrangements (Berend 2016; Jacobson 2016). In legal practice, intent has been used as a tiebreaker for collaborative reproduction when two different women have the gestational and genetic ties to a child and there is no other clear way to decide parentage (Dolgin 2000). This practice originated with the California Supreme Court's final reasoning in *Johnson v. Calvert* (1993), which sought to determine whether a gestational surrogate (Anna Johnson) had any parental rights to the child she had carried and given birth to. The child was conceived using an embryo created from the gametes of a married heterosexual couple (Mark and Crispina Calvert), who were ultimately intending to raise the child. Rather than relying on either gestation or genetics as the basis for maternity, the court creatively reasoned that the original intention to have the child came earlier in the process than either biological relationship and resided only with one woman (Calvert).

Bemoaning the lack of consistency and stability in court decisions related to collaborative reproduction, the legal scholar Linda Anderson (2009, 34) argued that using an intent-based test of parentage could provide legal predictability, lead to "reasonable results" for all involved parties, and accommodate rapidly changing technologies in postmodern family building. Although there has been little agreement in settling on a new paradigm for maternity determinations, one common critique raised by many legal scholars is that current methods are "fact-intensive" (Kindregan 2009, 621) and highly contextual (Dolgin 2000). Maternity has become a situational accomplishment as opposed to a taken-for-granted biolegal fact in the post-IVF era.

A Social Worlds and Arenas Approach

Addressing the conversations and conflicts about defining maternity is challenging and requires looking for places where these discussions are most likely to occur. I conceptualize reproductive medicine and law as distinct but interacting social worlds in the parentage and reproduction arena. Working from the symbolic interaction tradition in sociology, Anselm Strauss (1978, 121) described social worlds as "universes of discourse." These universes loosely define social actors who communicate and interact about specific substantive areas (e.g., childbirth, pregnancy, and parental rights). Strauss also argued for looking at social worlds as universes of practice, focusing on activities central to the world (e.g., research, therapy, and teaching); members and core actors or representatives; physical and virtual sites where activities take place (e.g., labs, clinics, offices, and conference halls), and various technologies (e.g., AI and IVF) and organizations (e.g., ethics committees) that are connected to or embedded in these worlds. In my usage here, 'discourse' refers broadly to shared communication and the tangible products or evidence of that communication, which both reflect and constitute social worlds (Gubrium and Holstein 1993; Strauss 1978). For instance, through concrete products like research articles, editorials, press releases, and committee reports, social world actors communicate ideas and information about their various activities to one another and to external worlds, but they also negotiate, implicitly or explicitly, the standards and jurisdiction of those activities.

The social worlds of reproductive medicine and law converge around particular issues related to collaborative reproduction, especially discussions about the morality and legality of reproductive technologies and about family building and parentage. This point of convergence is an arena of action or arena of concern where "multiple worlds [are] organized ecologically around issues of mutual concern and commitment to action" (Clarke and Star 2008, 113). In such arenas, individual representatives or professional bodies from each world come together to communicate, express conflicts, and sometimes foster mutual understanding or action toward a common goal.

Reproductive medicine is a recognized subfield of Western biomedicine. It has a set of central activities, including basic and applied research and clinical or therapeutic work. It has distinct technologies and techniques for carrying out the work (e.g., IVF, AID, egg donation, and gestational surrogacy). It also has recognizable professional organizations, notably the ASRM, which anchors the social world internally and externally represents its interests and members to others. Although I began my work on this project primarily by examining the social world of reproductive medicine, I quickly realized that other outside actors and organizations were often involved either structurally or discursively. Some external actors had formal roles as members of professional advisory committees in reproductive medicine. Others frequently published in *Fertility and Sterility*—the flagship journal for U.S. reproductive medicine, launched in 1950—thereby directing their communication at reproductive researchers and practitioners and sometimes acting as a liaison between the social world of reproductive medicine and various professional or regulatory bodies. In tracing the communications and activities of reproductive medicine, I also saw that legal uncertainty emerged early on as a primary concern in collaborative reproduction.

As a social world, law is more diffuse than reproductive medicine, even when it enters the arena of collaborative reproduction and parentage. I chose to focus on relatively bounded and concrete instances in which parentage issues emerged, such as court cases, statutes, legislative hearings, and debates. These meaning-making activities are conducted in smaller sites, but incrementally they have wide-reaching implications for families across the United States. Some of these activities are more top-down, like the development of the Uniform Parentage Act—a model act developed in the 1970s to clarify parent-child relations, which states can choose to adopt in part or in full (Uniform Law Commission [ULC] 2021a, 2021b, and 2021c). However, many activities are more decentralized, requiring immersion into the specific state or local contexts to understand what is happening on the ground. I aimed to balance both analytic levels.

An enduring methodological question is how to analyze social worlds (Clarke and Star 2008). One of my major strategies was to look for tangible products of communication and activities within and between reproductive medicine and law. I focused on central actors, such as those in leadership positions as journal editors or organizational presidents and notable scientists or practitioners making advances in the field. I also identified relevant committees, hearings, conferences, and organizations, using these as major nodes in mapping the social world activities. I relied on a range of documentary data sources that I collected for this project between 2012 and 2020, which I describe in greater detail in the chapter outlines below. I conducted all the content coding and analysis, using an "immersion/crystallization" strategy (Borkan 1999). During the first cycle of coding the data (Saldana 2009), I used a relatively open strategy, reading the various documents and marking passages that rose to the surface, sensitized by my driving research questions. After reviewing sets of documents related to an issue, I typically created memos with my observations and initial interpretations. Many of these formed the basis of later, more in-depth analyses. My coding approach involved both a priori codes based on previous research (codes such as genetics, gestation, and intent as the foundation of parenthood) and emerging codes. I looked for some stories (e.g., about gender and families), but I also let the data tell me other stories along the way that I had not anticipated.

Chapter Outline and Methods Overview

Over the next several chapters, I peer into the social worlds of U.S. reproductive medicine and law to look at different aspects of maternity as it is being (re)constructed as a medical and legal phenomenon in the post-IVF era. In chapter 2, I first take a quick tour through some ideas and definitions, thinking about the connections between maternity, mother, and mothering and offering the concept of the *repronormative family* to bridge different ideologies of family and kinship.

In chapter 3, I focus on how donor replacement of genetic parentage has different implications for paternity and maternity. Some of these differences are connected to the timeframes and reproductive politics of when AI and IVF—the two technologies that make sperm and egg donation, respectively, possible—first emerged. For instance, I show that these technologies were differently framed using a *politics of family* versus a *politics of life* approach. But I also argue that the different implications of donor gametes are further rooted in a gendered biological paradox: men are pre-sumed to easily part with (i.e., donate) their sperm but not to eas-ily receive other men's sperm, while women are presumed to easily receive other women's eggs but not to easily part with their own. My data sources for this chapter included clinical research, edito-rials, and other commentary from U.S. physicians at the center of the research on and practice of reproductive medicine during the emergence and uptake of sperm and egg donation. I relied on pub-lished reports and guidelines from professional bodies such as the American Fertility Society (AFS), previously known as the Amer-ican Society for the Study of Sterility (ASSS), and currently named the ASRM. I also included views of external actors who prominently intersected with this social world, such as by publish-ing commentaries in medical journals or acting as nonmedical advisory experts on professional committees. To get a sense of reproductive medicine in its early years, I relied on a 1994 "insider history" (to borrow a term from Clarke 1998, 277) of the first fifty years of the AFS, written by Walter Duka (a former editor and reporter at the *Washington Post*) and Alan DeCherney (then AFS president-elect and a professor in and chair of the Department of Obstetrics and Gynecology at Tufts University School of Medi-cine). I supplemented this with other works written by prominent physicians, sometimes in collaboration with outside experts (Cohen 1996; Crockin and Jones 2010; Leeton 2013; Sauer 1996). I also loosely tracked editorial conversations in *Fertility and Sterility* to get a sense of the pressing issues of the times. A former editor in chief, Roger Kempers (1980, 1), described the journal as the major "organ for the communication of scientific information . . . in the field of reproductive medicine." The "Editor's Corner" section was introduced in 1980 with the specific goal of providing practition-ers with content on social, legal, ethical, and religious issues related to fertility and assisted reproduction (Kempers 1980).

Fertility and Sterility provided a natural hub for more targeted data collection on professional and practitioner discussions of gam-ete donation. I began with citation searches using sets of key-words for each reproductive technique: "artificial insemination," "donor sperm," "AID," and "donor insemination," "donor egg/ovum/oocyte," and "egg/ovum/oocyte donation." I then relied on a snowball citation-tracking method (Greenhalgh and Peacock 2005) to broaden coverage and pick up additional articles by scanning the reference lists of each article. Sometimes this method took me beyond *Fertility and Sterility* to other prominent medical outlets such as the *Journal of the American Medical Association (JAMA)*, *New England Journal of Medicine (NEJM)*, and *American Journal of Obstetrics & Gynecology (AJOG)*. These outlets held early professional discourse on artificial insemination that predated the 1950 establishment of *Fertility and Sterility*. I used the selective snowball citation technique until I had achieved reasonable coverage through "saturation" (Morse 1995)—the point at which reference lists of the articles and reports I had found showed no new information that I deemed relevant to the specific topics at hand. I also made room for "serendipitous discovery" (Greenhalgh and Peacock 2005, 1064)—the act of finding something useful, informative, or thought provoking while searching for something else. My focused analysis of gamete donation in the second part of the chapter primarily relied on fifty articles addressing AID (starting in 1921, with most published in the 1950s–1970s); eighty-nine articles addressing egg donation (published in the 1980s–1990s), with some retrospective reflections published in the 2000s and edited volumes for additional context; and four significant reports published by the AFS Ethics Committee between 1984 and 1994.

In chapter 4, I move into a more contemporary timeframe (mid-2010s), analyzing literature developed for patients considering egg donation, embryo donation, and gestational surrogacy. I examine maternal claims-making in different forms of collaborative reproduction and introduce the concepts of *contingent maternity* and the *conjugal embryo*. I show how professional reproductive medicine helps infertile (heterosexual and partnered) women construct and justify their maternal claims through different claims-making pathways and strategies. These constructions are inherently at odds with one another—they perpetuate tensions between genetic or gestational and nature or nurture definitions of authentic maternity, depending on the intended audience and reproductive technique being discussed. Yet while this inherent tension focuses our attention on eggs versus wombs as the root of authentic maternity, it overlooks the contingent and situational aspects of post-IVF maternities, which require a constellation of factors to align for them to be fully recognized as maternity. I argue that contemporary reproductive medicine does not define maternity via collaborative reproduction as a truly autonomous maternal connection to a child. Instead, these forms of maternity are highly contingent and, therefore, potentially discreditable identities (Goffman 1963).

My early thinking about the analysis in this chapter came out of my dissertation and subsequent work in 2009–2012 on the U.S. fertility industry. I had previously collected hundreds of packets for gamete donors or recipients from clinics, agencies, and sperm banks across the country to examine clinic policies and the constructions of gamete donation practices. As I gathered these packets, I noticed that clinic material frequently included not just specific forms for the clinic but also copies of two commonly used booklets on egg donation. I recall sitting at my graduate student desk in a shared office poring over these booklets. My preliminary thoughts were that they were quite sympathetic to egg donation maternity, assuring women that the nurture of pregnancy outweighed the nature of genetics. I decided to pursue this analysis further and began to collect additional literature for patients to see how egg donation was represented, compared to gestational surrogacy and embryo donation. Having been immersed in studying the U.S. fertility industry, I knew that two key sources for patient literature were the ASRM and RESOLVE: The National Infertility Association. These organizations had public, digitized literature online. I downloaded all relevant literature and added the original two patient booklets to the analysis, collecting twenty-eight unique data sources in all.

In chapter 5, I address the social world of law as it grapples with collaborative reproduction and parentage. I do so by examining two embryo mix-up cases that went to court: *Perry-Rogers v. Fasano* (2000), and *Robert B. and Denise B. v. Susan B.* (2003). I use these cases to underscore the maternity uncertainty and legal ambiguity that comes with fragmenting maternity. I describe *maternity designation* as an important yet overlooked sociolegal process in contemporary motherhood theorizing. This process refers to the activity of sorting through and affirming or rejecting various maternal claims with the goal of assigning maternity to a specific person. The two cases I analyze also show how maternity is unequally constructed, especially considering race, biology, and marital status. Families that fall short of the repronormative paradigm are disrupted, invaded, and fear losing their rights to their children. Yet it is also challenging to articulate and solidify parental rights to a child who is yet to be born under conditions of fragmented and disembodied maternity.

I analyzed both court documents and media coverage of these two U.S. embryo mix-up cases. My initial interest in embryo mix-ups came from reading about cases in the United Kingdom and the Netherlands. Although these cases were not technically about intentional collaborative reproduction, I felt that they would create situations of unease and uncertainty that would contribute further to thinking about maternity in conflict. I also wanted to think through situations other than *In re Baby M* and *Johnson v. Calvert*—cases that formed early legal, social, and scholarly responses to fragmented maternity. And in my reading of the existing literature, IVF mix-ups seemed less prominently covered but just as full of controversy. I identified the two U.S. cases through a broad media search in *Access World News* using the search terms "IVF clinic" and "mix up." This initial search returned eighty-six unique articles, primarily covering the two cases. A third embryo mix-up involving the Savages and Morells also came up in the media coverage search but did not include legal action, so it does not appear in my comparative analysis later in the chapter. I began the analysis for this chapter thinking that I would focus primarily on U.S. media coverage, but I soon found that to be somewhat lacking as a sole data source. Wanting to think more about the dynamics of each case, I turned to the published court records in LexisNexis. This chapter ultimately offers a comparative case analysis. Although not really counterfactuals to one another, the two embryo mix-up cases help isolate certain variables about fragmented maternity (genetic, gestational, and social) and conditions of family inequality (related to marital status and race) and raise some important questions about maternity uncertainty and legal designation of parentage.

In chapter 6, I take up the question of legal regulation: how are states legislating intentionally fragmented maternities? I first briefly look at state-level statutory law on parentage and collaborative reproduction to provide an overall sketch of the regulatory landscape. I then conduct an in-depth case analysis of Louisiana law in 1986–2016 on IVF and collaborative reproduction. In 1986, Louisiana became the first state to address embryo donation parentage, but it spent the next three decades grappling with how to address other types of collaborative reproduction—producing a piecemeal and sometimes contradictory view of what constitutes maternity and parentage. Focusing on Louisiana gives a close-up view of the various debates and sense-making activities that happen during the legislative process.

I relied primarily on the LexisNexis database as my first stop for collecting data on legislative activities such as proposed bills, enacted or revised statutes, and state legal codes. I supplemented this with searching state legislative websites for digitized materials and requesting copies of archived documents to track bills through a legislative history method, collecting written records of bills being introduced and debated, résumé digests, house or senate journals, minutes, and voting records, as well as video files of different committees and legislative bodies discussing specific bills. For video files, I downloaded the files, clipped pertinent sections of committee meetings, and transcribed files to produce textual transcripts for later analysis. Although my main strategy for legislative data was to go right to the primary sources first, I also tracked down related media coverage and investigated the specific actors speaking in support or opposition, so I could understand the organizations or interests they represented.

In the concluding chapter, I return to the notion of maternity uncertainty. This uncertainty is part of the broader landscape of postmodern families—dismantling hegemonic ideologies of family and replacing those with diverse relationships and ways of forming those relationships. Deinstitutionalization creates space for recognizing a wider array of maternal-child relationships, but it is also plagued by a lack of social and legal protection. Thus, I argue that maternity in the post-IVF era is an incomplete institution, lacking consensus, guiding norms, and institutional support.

2

Conceiving Motherhood and the Repronormative Family

What does maternity mean? Being a mother? Mothering? Before turning to my empirical analysis, I want to take a brief tour through the idea of maternity and the relationship between maternity, mother, and mothering. Colloquially, the term "maternity" appears in a few different contexts. Maternity care is a medical subspecialty focusing on prenatal care and pregnancy. Maternal and child health is an arena of health care that recognizes the interdependence between two people, or between a pregnant person and a child-to-be. These uses of "maternity" all refer to the embodied and actual, or expected, relationship between a woman and a fetus or child. "Maternal" also refers to the qualities of a relationship or a behavior. People can act in maternal ways—specifically, nurturing (or mothering) ways—toward another person.

In Western culture, we often conflate maternity, mothering, and mother. They collapse into one another. The biological and embodied relationship is assumed to provide the foundation for the nurturing behavior. This biosocial linkage becomes apparent through the themes of nesting, nurturing, and preparing that pervade discussions of pregnancy and subsequent motherhood. A prominent maternity nursing textbook from the 1970s describes the changing uterine lining, anticipating pregnancy, as "preparing a nesting place for the ovum . . . should it be fertilized" (Hamilton

1971, 22). The American Pregnancy Association's website (2021) devotes a page to nesting and pregnancy, questioning not the "instinct" itself but the "old wives' tale" that the instinct indicates the start of labor: "the overwhelming desire to get your home ready for your new baby. The nesting instinct is strongest in the later weeks. . . . It is an old wives' tale that once nesting urges begin, labor is about to come on. . . . Nesting is common and is considered to be an instinct to prepare for birth, but not all pregnant women experience the nesting instinct." The page features an image of a white woman dusting her kitchen cabinets, cheerfully smiling at onlookers, and anticipating labor and new motherhood. A recent edition of *The Womanly Art of Breastfeeding*—a now-classic book developed by early La Leche League members—introduces breast-feeding as "more than just a way to feed your baby. It's the way you're naturally designed to begin your mothering experience" (Wiessinger, West, and Pitman 2010, 5). In the first chapter, titled "Nesting," the authors address the imagined pregnant woman reading the book: "You're 'nesting'—gathering the things your baby will need and making a place for him in your home. . . . But while you're out shopping, your body is quietly preparing the real 'nest' . . . your breasts. . . . [Your baby's] go-to place for warmth, security, comfort, love, and yes, food" (5). Cisgender women gestate, give birth, and experience that wash of postpartum hormones. The biological process prepares them for motherhood, whether they realize it or not. To give birth is to bring this process to fruition, to become a mother. Maternal instincts kick in and ensure ultimate devotion to, and care for, one's biological child. So the story goes.

The concepts "maternity," "mother," and "mothering" also appear in biological, social-psychological, and legal realms of study. The maternal-child dyad is widely recognized in biological and child development research as a primary human bond. In their now-classic work on maternal-infant bonding, the prominent pediatricians Marshall H. Klaus and John H. Kennell (1976, 1) argued: "Perhaps the mother's attachment to her child is the strongest bond in the human." Though typically defined and understood as a social relationship, the maternal-child bond is also associated with the series of neuroendocrine and sensory changes that occur during late pregnancy, parturition, and the postpartum period (Broad, Curley, and Keverne 2006; Maestripieri 2001; Purhonen et al. 2001). In these contexts, however, there are both more arguments and more evidence that giving birth is neither necessary nor sufficient for prompting mothering behavior—unlike the dominant cultural stories we tell. In attempting to "unravel the mysteries of maternal attachment," Klaus and Kennell (1976, 3) addressed the counterfactual: the cases in which women, and other female primates and mammals (e.g., rats) did not bond with the infants they gave birth to, what they described as "mothering disorders." Perhaps even more mysterious and intriguing, Klaus and Kennell also identified those cases in which "virgin" (i.e., non-parturient) female animals and male animals engaged in mothering behaviors with young (1976, 32). Based on this varied evidence, Klaus and Kennell (1976, 31) argued for recognizing a "sensitive period" directly after birth during which maternal-infant bonding is most successful and specifically applied this to human attachment. Any separation and disturbance during this "sensitive period" could have long-lasting effects on the maternal-child bond.[1] Klaus and Kennell's bonding hypothesis has been substantially critiqued (D. Eyer 1994), but it also made a strong case for the idea that giving birth did not always cause women to act maternally toward their babies. It was not a guarantee.

Feminist scholars have also spent a lot of time critiquing the assumption that giving birth is a necessary or sufficient condition for maternal behavior, aiming to decouple the biological and the social in women's lives. In *The Future of Motherhood*, the sociologist Jessie Bernard (1974, 19) described the "biological substrate" of motherhood, noting that "the first imperative of motherhood . . . is to reproduce." Bernard further argued that it was over this "biological substrate" that lay the patriarchal ideas about motherhood that were so damaging to women. Much feminist attention has since turned to the social and cultural, to de-essentialize motherhood and uncouple womanhood from motherhood. To this end, many have argued that we should focus on mothering to understand how "biological [reproductive] activities are culturally organized" (Arendell 2000, 1193). Feminist research points to examples such as cross-cultural differences in expectations for mother-child relationships (Collier, Rosaldo, and Yangisako 1992) and addresses issues such as postpartum depression (Taylor 1996) and infanticide (Gordon 1976) that violate the seemingly natural romanticized bond between mother and child. Other research addresses the process of becoming a mother, showing how women transition into maternal identities rather than instantly and instinctually being or feeling like mothers by virtue of having given birth (Mercer 2004). Yet most of this research still assumes that pregnancy and childbirth are precursors to women's maternal identity transition and social definition as mothers. What happens when we remove biology?

Research on nonnormative motherhoods exposes the ideological hierarchy according to which biological motherhood—along with the expectation of raising one's own children—is privileged over purely social motherhood (Letherby 1999; Wegar 1998). Studies of lesbian co-parents, adoptive mothers, and stepmothers underscore tensions that arise in legitimating maternal identities without a biological relationship. Lesbian motherhood is often invisible or inconceivable in normative understandings of reproduction and parenthood (Agigian 2004; Mamo 2007), but lesbian "co-mothers" who do not have any biological connection to their child may particularly exist in a "legal . . . social and emotional netherworld" (Muzio 1993, 225). Their parental relationship to the child has typically been defined indirectly, through their relationship with the biological mother. Prior to the marriage equality decision by the U.S. Supreme Court in *Obergefell v. Hodges* (2015), nonbiological co-mothers had little recourse in claiming legal parentage other than through second-parent adoption (having to adopt their own child or children) or being recognized as a de facto parent (Nejaime 2021). The sociologist Nancy Naples (2004, 681) describes these indirect pathways to parentage, especially having to adopt one's own child, as "reinscrib[ing] the nonbiological co-mother's otherness." Research on stepmothers' experiences suggests that women define themselves as mothering but distinctly not being the mother of their stepchildren (Weaver and Coleman 2005). These scenarios emphasize the centrality of the biological mother and the marginality of the co-mother and stepmother.

Studies of adoptive parenting suggest that both men and women believe that women's so-called maternal instinct will engage for women with adoptive children (Miall and March 2003). Yet birth mothers do not lose their claim to maternity by not raising their biological children. They may be culturally defined as "bad" mothers (Wegar 1997), but they are still granted some form of sociolegal recognition as a mother by virtue of having given birth. This is evidenced by the fact that in thirty-three states, there is a waiting period after birth (anywhere from twelve hours to fifteen days) before birth mothers can officially give consent for their child to be adopted (Child Welfare Information Gateway 2021). Furthermore, birth mothers might be able to revoke that consent within a certain period (which varies from state to state), recognizing their possible desire to mother the children they gave birth to. Additionally, although adoption is an intuitive solution to involuntary childlessness resulting from infertility and other causes, many people view adoption as "second best" in the "reproductive hierarchy" of options (Bell 2019, 480 and 483). The sociologist Ann Bell (2019) points to how the medicalization of infertility has served to reinforce the biological kinship ideal, subordinating adoptive parenthood to efforts to achieve biological parenthood with infertility treatments.

Feminist scholarship addressing racial or ethnic variations in mothering has identified "othermothers," using an Afrocentric perspective on Black women and motherhood (Hill Collins 1990, 119). Othermothers help "bloodmothers" with child-care responsibilities and "traditionally have been central to the institution of Black motherhood" (119). The sociologist Dawn Marie Dow (2016) more recently described this as one part of an alternate ideology of motherhood that her Black interviewees espoused, which she referred to as "integrated mothering." The concept of othermothers broadens the notion of who is responsible for mothering and is directly juxtaposed with the dominant ideology of an exclusive mothering relationship between one mother and her child or children (Bernard 1974; Hays 1996). Yet the original concepts of blood-mother and othermother still root the initial mother in blood or biology, without which the distinction would be unnecessary.

Scholars of infertility and assisted or collaborative reproduction have had to grapple much more directly with blocked or challenged pathways to achieving fully integrated biosocial maternity. Arthur Greil (1991), Margarete Sandelowski (1993), and Gay Becker (2000) all poignantly conveyed how the experience of infertility and involuntary childlessness threatens normative, gendered pathways for adulthood and challenges the expectation that so-called normal women should easily become pregnant when they desire. Bell's (2014) more recent work added insights into how infertility, as a highly medicalized phenomenon in the United States, is differentially experienced by women of lower socioeconomic status. Bell argued that women of lower socioeconomic status who also have infertility are doubly marginalized and "must challenge two dominant stereotypes . . . [that] all women are mothers . . . [and that] all infertile women are higher class" (2014, 57). Other scholars have focused more on how specific assisted or collaborative reproductive technologies challenge or reinforce cultural conceptions of motherhood (for good or for bad). In *Recreating Motherhood*, Barbara Katz Rothman (1989, 23) argued that motherhood was being transformed from older (harmful) definitions as an all-encompassing status for women to newer (also harmful) definitions of motherhood as "an activity . . . service . . . work . . . and children as the product." Surrogacy, according to Rothman, was one such example of how motherhood was being redefined, but in ways that reflected hegemonic patriarchal (egg = woman's seed), capitalist (baby = product), and technological (bodies = machines) ideologies as opposed to those emphasizing nurturance, care, and connection. The sociologist Susan Markens addressed the emergence and framing of surrogacy as a social problem, examining the culture wars over surrogacy as a moral solution for infertile couples versus an immoral practice akin to baby selling. Markens argued that the debate about surrogacy reflected deeper "concerns ... [about] the meaning of motherhood and ... the future of white families" (2007, 8). Surrogacy's emergence as a social problem offered a symbolic site upon which these discussions can play out. Given that surrogacy challenges hegemonic gender and family ideologies and potentially casts surrogates as deviant, especially vis-à-vis their own families, later work by Zsuzsa Berend (2016), Elizabeth Ziff (2017), and Heather Jacobson (2021) importantly shows how surrogates actively manage surrogacy as a moral project, aligning with notions of altruistic self-sacrifice, duty, and responsibility.

Focusing more directly on questions of kinship and maternity in collaborative reproduction, the anthropologist Elly Teman's (2010, 110) work on Israeli surrogates showed how both surrogates and intended mothers simultaneously downplayed the role of the surrogate while emphasizing the intended mother through the work of "maternal-claiming." Teman defined the latter as "techniques aimed at claiming entitlement to the social label of mother of the expected baby" (110). In her broader analysis of the labor of surrogacy, Jacobson, a sociologist, found that many U.S.-based surrogates were reluctant to work with intended mothers who were not using their own eggs because their insecurities about maternity created "an extra layer of [emotional] labor" (2016, 90) for surrogates to manage during the journey. Addressing both egg donation and surrogacy in the United States Charis Thompson, a science and technology studies scholar, identified "relational" versus "custodial" stages of reproduction (2005, 148). Thompson defined the former stage as one that "can support claims of parenthood," while the latter "involve[s] caring for the gametes or embryos ... [and] cannot sustain parental claims" (148). These different conceptual stages help "disambiguate" kinship between collaborative actors, especially in cases using intrafamilial donors and surrogates (145). The sociologist Amrita Pande's (2009) work on gestational surrogacy in India addressed how surrogates claimed kinship to a surrogate-born child through the shared bodily substances of blood (nourishment through gestation), sweat (from the labor of gestation), and breast milk (if a surrogate did the breast-feeding). Yet Pande distinctly identified these ties as a type of "everyday forms of kinship" that ultimately did not disturb the intended mother's sole maternity claim to the surrogacy-born child (2009, 393).

Addressing how surrogates themselves interpret and construct the "moral project" of surrogacy, Berend, a sociologist, offers additional insights into how U.S.-based surrogates view their relationships both to the "surro-babies" they help create and the intended parents that they go on surrogacy "journeys" with (2016, 11 and 59). Surrogates framed bonding and emotional attachment (to the intended parents as a couple or to the intended mother specifically) as important aspects of the surrogacy journey but also engaged in "kinship reorientations" to how they thought about the surro-baby as being the intended parents' baby from the start—a baby "conceived in the heart" (79 and 74). Pregnancy was a necessary but insufficient condition to make someone a mother. Some surrogates might "play mommy" (79) on occasion to a surro-baby, but only if there was no intended mother in the family constellation—for example, if they were a surrogate for a single man or a gay male couple. Even with traditional surrogacy (where the surrogate contributes both egg and gestation), Berend noted that surrogates framed the practice as "giving a piece of yourself" but distinctly not as giving up "their own children" (78). Some traditional surrogates, Berend noted, thought of surro-babies as part of their extended family constellation but never as members of their nuclear family, drawing careful boundaries between their own family and the intended parents' family.

The existing research on infertility and collaborative reproduction gives us glimpses into the different types of family and kinship conundrums that various actors (donors, surrogates, and intended parents) must work through in creating families. I build on this existing work but zoom in more closely on the dilemma of fragmented maternity. I also look at the maternity dilemma as one that plays out not just interpersonally among the reproductive actors, but also in and through organizations, social worlds, and institutions. In examining fragmented maternity, we also need to conceptually parse out the biological, social, and legal elements of motherhood and not conflate maternity, mother, and mothering. To view these as separate but related elements of motherhood, I borrow from Candace West and Don Zimmerman's (1987) seminal work on "doing gender." Other feminist and family studies scholars have found the notion of "doing" to be conceptually helpful in the context of family and kinship (e.g., Nelson 2006; Thompson 2005). I find it useful for explicating the concepts of maternity, mother, and mothering. To avoid reducing sex and gender into one another, West and Zimmerman offered a three-part framework: sex, sex category, and (doing) gender. They identified sex as a "determination" arising from applying "socially agreed upon . . . criteria," and from this, an individual is placed in a sex category as a man or woman (1987, 127). Finally, an individual engages in "doing gender" as behavior that both emerges from norms to adhere to and bolsters their position in their specific sex category. In this vein, maternity, mother, and mothering represent interacting but distinct components of the institution of motherhood (Table 2.1). They do not have to reside in only one individual. Aiming to underscore the social construction of motherhood, feminist scholarship has emphasized mothering as behavior (akin to "doing gender") and mother as a social category and internalized identity (akin to sex category) but has done little analysis of maternity (a social determination akin to sex).

In this study, I use the following working definitions. Maternity refers to the assignment and recognition of a specific parental relationship between a woman and a child. Culturally, it refers to and privileges biology, but it also requires legitimation by the state for authenticity. Mother is both a social category and an internalized identity. Here I am drawing on Patricia Martin (2004) and Adrienne Rich (1986) to move away from viewing mother as a role, as well as to recognize mother as both an institutional status and an internalized identity based on personal experience. The concept of mother often assumes that biological maternity has been established, but it can also refer to a purely legal or socio-psychological relationship to a child. Mothering is the activity of nurturing and

TABLE 2.1 Analogous Frameworks of Gender
and Motherhood

Sex (assignment)		Maternity (designation)
Applying socially agreed upon biological criteria to categorize bodies as male or female	=	Sorting through, affirming, or rejecting various maternal claims with the goal of assigning maternity to a person or persons
Sex category Emerging social and personal identity as man or woman	=	Mother Emerging social and personal identity in relation to self and child
Doing gender Situational conduct held "accountable" to "normative conceptions" of masculinity and femininity" (West and Zimmerman 1987, 136).	=	Mothering Behaviors and practices related to child rearing and their normative evaluation, which varies across time and place

caring for another individual (Glenn, Chang, and Forcey 1994). It requires neither maternity nor social or legal recognition as a mother. Indeed, many women engage in mothering activities but are not formally recognized as a mother of a given child (Hequembourg 2004; MacDonald 2010; Weaver and Coleman 2005). For my purposes here, I am primarily interested in maternity, but maternity definitions and decisions spill over into who gets to take the baby home, is recognized as that baby's mother, and subsequently does the daily work of mothering.

Questions about maternity and motherhood are just one piece of family and kinship: they also interact with broader ideologies about who and what constitutes a family. Throughout my analysis I develop and use the concept of the repronormative family as shorthand for a more complex ideological package. I offer the concept as a combination and extension of existing feminist scholarship about hegemonic family and kinship ideologies and the feminist legal concept of repronormativity. Drawing these literatures together, the concept of the repronormative family conveys ideas about what families should look like in form and function, as well as how they should be created.

The view of maternity as a biosocial, exclusive, and enduring relationship to a child is integral to hegemonic cultural ideas about the Western family more broadly. Historical analyses show that these specific cultural ideas first appeared in the late eighteenth and early nineteenth centuries. Describing dominant child-rearing norms in Europe in the Middle Ages, the sociologist Sharon Hays (1996, 23) noted that children were considered unruly, "demonic creatures" and child rearing was seen as an "onerous task . . . certainly there was no belief in a maternal instinct that led mothers to protect and nurture their young." Rather, women were often tasked with child rearing because it was menial work, not because of their presumed natural abilities. However, such views about children and child rearing began to be transformed in the seventeenth and eighteenth centuries. By the nineteenth century, childhood was largely understood as a period of innocence rather than one of original sin, and mothers took on a greater and more direct role in child rearing, based on the assumption that the mother-child dyad had a unique, affective relationship within the family (Hays 1996; Pleck 1998). One example that reflects this cultural shift is the 'tender years doctrine' that increasingly influenced custody decisions from the early nineteenth century until the mid-twentieth century. Fathers initially had exclusive rights of and obligations for child custody after marital dissolution—something that early feminists fought against in articulating women's marital and familial rights (Flexner 1975; Pleck 1998). By contrast, the tender years doctrine emphasized the unique need that young children, especially those under the age of seven, had to be placed in maternal custody (Hyde 1984a and 1984b). Addressing the history of this development, the legal scholar Laurance Hyde (1984a, 2) observed: "With the Industrial Revolution shifting the father's workplace from the farm to the office and factory, the world suddenly discovered woman's maternal instincts. Although she had always been at home with the children, for the first time her husband was not peering over her shoulder."

While cultural ideas about (white, middle-class) parent-child relations were changing, so were ideas about (white, middle-class) marriage and the domestic division of labor. Bernard (1981) described this as the emergence of a particular structure of the so-called traditional family and complementary, gendered roles of the good provider and the housewife. Although Bernard purported to document the rise and fall of the good-provider role from approximately 1830 to 1980, more than a decade later, the sociologist Dorothy Smith (1993, 52) described a variant of this role in the ideology of the Standard North American Family (SNAF): "It is a conception of the family as a legally married couple sharing a household. The adult male is in paid employment. . . . The adult female may also earn an income, but her primary responsibility is the care of husband, household, and children." SNAF, Smith argued, was like a form of cultural DNA: a universalizing "ideological code . . . that replicates its organization in multiple and various sites" (51). The legal scholar Martha Fineman (1993) similarly observed that the heterosexual nuclear family exists as a venerated and naturalized family form in the law and other social institutions. The traditional family ideal had not met its demise—it was still lurking as a standard with which to compare alternative family forms. As the sociologist Margaret Andersen (1991, 236) noted, "in the face of structural changes, the traditional family ideal no longer describes actual family experiences—if, indeed, it ever did. Yet data on beliefs and behavior indicate that people still hold to the ideal. . . . [I]deals persist despite vast structural changes."

Biological reproduction is a central component of dominant ideals and narratives of the family. In this vein, the family ideal works in tandem with a kinship ideal that the "genetic family . . . [is] the most central social unit. . . . [Genetic] connection . . . implies a sense of belonging, continuity, and care that makes families—and society—possible" (Wegar 1998, 41). Compared to the kinship ideal, other forms of familial connections are interpreted as secondary, not creating a real family. These two ideals are confronted head-on in assisted and collaborative reproduction, where intended parents might have to compromise on the kinship ideal to preserve some of the vestiges of the family ideal.

The concept of repronormativity further highlights the linkages between the family and kinship ideals. The feminist legal scholar Katherine Franke (2001, 187) first described repronormativity as a compulsory "maternalization of female identity," akin to compulsory heterosexuality (Rich 1980). To be a woman was to inevitably be (or become) maternal: "Repronormative forces affect women's child-bearing and raising 'choices,' just as (hetero)sexuality has come to be understood as both compulsory and ineluctably the product of heteronormative forces" (Franke 2001, 197). Importing Franke's concept into queer and trans legal theorizing, Lara Karaian (2013) and Anna Weissman (2017) further developed repronormativity to refer to cultural ideas that underscore reproduction as a natural, inevitable function of the heteropatriarchal family. The stories of heteromasculinity and heterofemininity are also reproductive narratives. Heterosexual women become pregnant and give birth. They become mothers and mother children. Heterosexual men impregnate women through procreative sex. They father children and become fathers. And in the name of legitimacy and state-sanctioned reproductive acts, this happens within the monogamous marital family. All of these ideals and ideas come together in the notion of the repronormative family.

On its surface, the repronormative family clearly refers to (cis) gender and (hetero)sexuality. It also invokes race and class and other social inequalities, by broadly categorizing people as "legitimate or illegitimate reproducer[s]" (Weissman 2017, 280). In *Queering Reproduction* (2007, 59), the sociologist Laura Mamo described how lesbian women are culturally positioned as the "nonreproductive other" relative to heterosexual women's assumed default status as procreative. The legal scholar Lisa Ikemoto (1996) similarly argued that assisted reproductive technologies created three distinct stories about reproduction: the infertile, the "too fertile," and the "dysfertile." The "too fertile" story focuses on groups whose fertility and sexuality are labeled deviant: "unwed adult women, teens, welfare recipients, and/or women of color" (1008). The "dysfertile" story addresses gay men and lesbian women—invisible, marginalized, and nonprocreative. Juxtaposed with both, the "infertile" story includes those who are socially and culturally at the center: white, heterosexual, and married, but needing procreative assistance. Ideas about repronormativity and the imagined "boundaries of use" of assisted reproduction (Ikemoto 1996, 1009) perpetuate what the anthropologist Shellee Colen (1995) described as "stratified reproduction." The concept of stratified reproduction recognizes how certain family forms and family-building routes are empowered and viewed as natural, while others are disempowered and denaturalized.

Natural does not always mean biological. It can also refer to what is considered "good, moral, and inevitable" (Dolgin 1997, 115). While the repronormative family overwhelmingly invokes biological kinship through both shared genetics and maternal gestation, it also relies on a moral order of the traditional family ideal. This distinction helps make sense of how certain natural (genetic or gestational) bonds might be downplayed in favor of a more natural (socially fit) family structure. For instance, Ricki Solinger's (1994, 288 and 290) historical work on unwed pregnancy in the United States showed how white unwed mothers were differently stigmatized: first by views on the "biology of illegitimacy"—according to which having a nonmarital birth would permanently mark the baby with "biological and moral ruin"—and later by psychological explanations that focused on the "neurotic unmarried mother." The latter paradigm advocated for separating the birth mother and child, placing the child for adoption with a family deemed to be more socially 'fit' (white, married, and middle class). Solinger observed (1994, 290): "For the first time, it took more than a baby to make a white girl or woman into a mother. Without a preceding marriage, a white female could not achieve true motherhood." The idea that some family structures are more natural than others is a continuous undercurrent of public and professional discourse on collaborative reproduction.[2] Over the next few chapters I use these various conceptual insights to explore a newly uncertain maternity that is either partially or wholly unmoored from a taken-for-granted biological bedrock.

3

Losing My Genetics

Paternal versus Maternal Concerns

As social institutions, motherhood and fatherhood are intimately bound up with gender and (hetero)sexuality. When I teach courses on gender or family, I ask my students what it means "to father" versus "to mother" a child. Though this may be a cliché, it is an effective discussion starter. My students often respond that fathering means to contribute your genetics to a child, impregnate someone, or act as the progenitor. Occasionally, they mention instilling values, providing for children economically, or disciplining their unruly behavior. Sometimes the students mention pregnancy and birth as part of mothering, but more often they talk about caring for children, physically and emotionally. If we take this at face value, biology is central to fatherhood but marginal to motherhood. However, the opposite has been codified into legal definitions: paternity is inferred conceptually, whereas maternity is observed physically (Delaney 1986). Paternity, closely associated with impregnation, is also sexualized, while maternity is asexualized (Earle 2003; Franke 2001; Gordon 1976). This reflects broader cultural beliefs about men's and women's reproductive behavior, which are also evident in evolutionary and psychoanalytic thought (Benedek 1960; Chodorow 1978; Deutsch 1991; Lorber and Moore 2006).

In 1875, the American feminist Antoinette Blackwell first published *The Sexes throughout Nature*,[1] in which she argued for men's and women's natural equality resulting from their complementary differentiation. Blackwell noted that women's "direct" responsibility for nurturing offspring translated into a greater natural capacity for "parental [maternal] love" while men's indirect nurturing meant that they did not need to develop as much "parental love" but that they had a greater natural capacity for "sexual love" (1973, 361 and 365). Monogamous, heterosexual pairing, according to Blackwell, would bring these "loves" together in a complementary, sexual division of labor. Nearly a century later, the prominent psychoanalyst Therese Benedek[2] addressed the human "reproductive drive," arguing that men's variant of this drive was to spread their "seed" as much as possible: their reproductive function was "discharged in one act, the aim of which is to deposit semen in the vagina" (1960, 1). In contrast, women's reproductive drive had more stages after the initial procreative act and involved filling their wombs; demanding exclusive investment from their reproductive partner (and family breadwinner); and focusing on fulfillment through gestating, birthing, and raising children. Similar ideas filtered into functional perspectives on the family in sociological scholarship. The sociologists Talcott Parsons and Robert Bales (1956) conceptualized the nuclear family as having two main functional roles: an instrumental, active (masculine) role oriented toward the outer or public world external to the family unit, and an expressive, passive (feminine) role oriented toward the domestic or private world of the family. According to these culturally differentiated ideas about gender and parenthood, infertility poses a distinctly gendered identity threat to the men and women who experience it (Becker 2000; Greil 1991). As the sociologist Liberty Walther Barnes (2014, 4–5) described in her book on masculinity and male infertility, "the ideal macho man is . . . virile and potent . . . [able to] get the sex he wants and impregnate a woman when he so desires. . . . Male infertility destabilizes [this ideal] . . . and hits personal masculine identities right where it counts." For women, on the other hand, infertility threatens their achievement of ideal womanhood and femininity in a pronatalist culture: their ability to become biological mothers (Letherby 1999; Sandelowski 1993).

In this chapter, I explore how these cultural ideas about biological parenthood, gender, and sexuality are woven through gamete donation. If fathering is largely associated with the (hetero) sexual procreative act, what happens when men use donor sperm to become fathers? If mothering is primarily associated with nurturance and care, does it matter if a woman uses a donor egg to conceive and bear a child? Egg and sperm donation are substantially more comparable reproductive scenarios than childbirth or surrogacy, which asymmetrically involve women's bodies much more than men's. They are also conceptually equivalent in what they aim to do: assist conception in which the gamete donor does not intend to have a legal or social relationship to the donor-conceived child (Englert et al. 2004). And as I show below, the technologies that made gamete donation possible—AI and IVF—were both met with strong reactions from the medical, legal, and religious worlds. Yet sociologists have found it both necessary and fruitful to analyze gamete donation with a gender lens (Almeling 2011; Haimes 1993b; Hertz, Nelson, and Kramer 2015; Johnson 2017a). The anthropologist Emily Martin (1991) showed how gametes culturally represent the microessences of masculinity and femininity: gender is distilled down to the cellular level. In this vein, I show that there are different meanings attached to paternal versus maternal genetics, creating distinct, gendered concerns about replacing parental gametes in the repronormative family.

To examine gendered concerns about genetic parentage, I move back in time to the emergence and popular uptake of gamete donation, first looking at AI and IVF. Professional actors in reproductive medicine are in conversation with those in other social worlds—especially law, religion, and other domains of medicine and science. I show that although there were many similarities in cultural reception (e.g., backlash) to the two technologies, they were also framed quite differently in terms of their social implications. AI discussions centered on a politics of family, whereas IVF discussions centered on a politics of life.

In the second part of the chapter, "Making Sense of Gamete Donation," I focus on how physicians in reproductive medicine professionally reckoned with the growing demand for AID and IVF. During the emergence of AID (in the 1920s–1950s), many medical and nonmedical professionals saw paternity as an urgent social problem. Who was the rightful, legal father of a donor-conceived child? Would men accept donor-conceived children as their own or reject them for lack of a genetic connection? The emergence of egg donation did not cause the same degree or type of concern for maternity. Both physicians and other experts and commentators seemed relatively untroubled about women's maternity via donor eggs. When it came to the donors, however, this pattern was reversed. Physicians paid minimal attention to sperm donors' motivations and experiences in the early decades of AID. They focused primarily on perpetuating a façade of biological paternity and having the sperm donor fade into the background. In egg donation, however, physicians were more suspicious of, and concerned about, women who were willing to donate their eggs—especially for nonfamilial donations. Some of this difference between sperm and egg donation, I argue, is due to preoccupation with other, pressing concerns, both inside and outside of reproductive medicine. These concerns centered on abortion politics and the status of the pre-embryo, and they threatened IVF research and therapy. Yet we cannot ignore the gendering of gametes and gamete donation as a social practice. Therefore, I also show how some of the difference in understanding egg versus sperm donation is framed by a gendered, biological paradox: genetic connections are simultaneously highly significant and utterly insignificant for both paternity and maternity.

Situating Assisted Reproduction

As therapeutic techniques to address infertility, AI and IVF emerged and gained popularity at different times during the twentieth century in the United States (Table 3.1). They were influenced not only by the different reproductive politics of their eras but also by changing models of physician-patient relationships (Daniels and Golden 2004; Kluchin 2011; Marsh and Ronner 1996; Thompson 2005).

TABLE 3.1 Situating AI and IVF Techniques

	AI	IVF
Emergence and popular uptake	1920s–1950s	1970s–1980s
Defined as mainstream	1970s	1990s
Physician-patient relations	Physician paternalism	Patient rights, informed consent; consumer oriented
Reproductive politics	Eugenics and birth control movements	Contraception and abortion rights, women's movement

One common historical backdrop was the shortage of white, native-born infants and young children for permanent adoption. The concept of 'sentimental adoption'—the notion that parents would adopt an infant or younger child to raise as their own, as opposed to an older child who might contribute more practically to the family—increasingly became a socially acceptable solution for involuntary childlessness in the early twentieth century (Marsh and Ronner 1996; Zelizer 1985). White, childless, married couples were particularly viewed as ideal adoptive parents because two social problems (unintended nonmarital pregnancy and involuntary childlessness) could be solved simultaneously (Marsh and Ronner 1996; Solinger 1994). But, as Margaret Marsh and Wanda Ronner (1996, 127) observed in their historical analysis of American infertility, "the demand for children under the age of five who were legally available for permanent adoption far outran the supply. . . . [A]doptive fervor did not abate in the 1920s, nor did the supply of adoptable babies become greater. Adoption alone could never solve . . . involuntary childlessness."

During the twentieth century, the social problem of involuntary childlessness was transformed into the medical problem of infertility. The sociologist Arthur Greil (1991, 41) noted that the development of reproductive endocrinology as a specialty produced a "watershed in the history of the medicalization. . . . Once they understood the menstrual cycle, physicians wasted little time in attempting to use this knowledge to regulate conception, pregnancy, and menopause."

As a result of such developments, more (white, middle-class) married couples turned to reproductive medicine to treat their fertility problems, using various therapeutic techniques. Yet all of these developments in understanding women's reproductive cycles and problems did little to address cases involving intractable male infertility. For that, the most promising technique was to bypass, as opposed to cure, the root cause by using assisted reproduction.[3]

AI was the earliest type of medically assisted reproduction and came in two forms: using the husband's sperm, or using donor sperm (AID). Physicians recommended using donor sperm in the cases of heterosexual couples in which the husband had severe male factor infertility, couples who had hereditary diseases that made it unwise to use their own gametes, and spouses with discordant Rh status.[4] Despite a long history of experimentation with humans dating back to the 1700s, physicians did not regularly practice any form of artificial insemination until the early to mid-twentieth century (Ombelet and Van Robays 2015). During the first half of the twentieth century infertility was largely constructed as a gynecological issue. Men were much less willing to be medically examined than their wives. Many physicians did not recognize or discuss male factors contributing to infertility. Those who did were unlikely to inform or openly treat men, to protect their masculine sensibilities (Almeling 2011; Barnes 2014; Marsh and Ronner 1996). For instance, semen analysis, which is simpler and physically less invasive than many procedures for testing female infertility, was not a regular part of the infertility work-up until the 1950s (Research Correlating Committee of the American Society for the Study of Sterility 1951). This slowly changed, as infertile couples increasingly requested AID. In a 1941 article in the *Journal of the American Medical Association (JAMA),* two New York-based physicians, Frances Seymour and Alfred Koerner, reported on a survey of AI sponsored by the National Research Foundation for the Eugenic Alleviation of Sterility. They estimated that 1,000–1,200 U.S. infants were being conceived annually using AI and that approximately one-third of those conceptions used donor sperm. Just a few decades later, Dr. Jerome Sherman (1973, 401)—an anatomist at the University of Arkansas Medical School working on

semen freezing and banking—observed that "thousands of inseminations have been performed with resounding success" and that AID
was deemed "a widely accepted medical practice."

Artificial insemination was a well-established infertility therapy when the first IVF baby was born in the late 1970s. IVF's history had started many decades earlier. Notably, John Rock and
Miriam Menkin (1944)[5] published an article on the first successful IVF experiment involving human eggs. However, it was not
until 1978 that the world's first IVF baby, Louise Brown, was born
in the United Kingdom (Duka and DeCherney 1994; Marsh and
Ronner 1996). Three years later, Drs. Howard and Georgeanna
Jones and colleagues at the Eastern Virginia Medical School oversaw the birth of the first IVF baby in the United States. As a
husband-wife team, known for both individual and joint excellence
in their scientific contributions, Drs. Howard and Georgeanna
Jones were both major figures in U.S. reproductive medicine and
figured prominently in the American Fertility Society (AFS): they
were early members, and later each assumed the role of president.
After retiring as faculty members from the Johns Hopkins University in 1978, they opened the first IVF center in the United States
in Norfolk, Virginia, the Jones Institute for Reproductive Medicine. The AFS newsletter hailed their 1981 IVF success as "a proud
moment for American medicine" (quoted in Duka and Decherney
1994, 165). Clinicians later described IVF as "forever alter[ing] the
treatment of infertility" (May and Hanshew 1990, 292).

IVF paved the way for other reproductive techniques: egg donation, embryo donation, and gestational surrogacy. These other
techniques relied on the ability to retrieve, externally manipulate,
and transfer reproductive cells back into or between women's
bodies for implantation and gestation. This newfound mobility of
gametes and embryos opened up incredible possibilities for medical
therapies as well as understanding reproductive processes through
basic research. Dr. Alan DeCherney, director of Reproductive
Endocrinology in the Department of Obstetrics and Gynecology
at Yale University, and then editor of *Fertility and Sterility*, described
the "exhilarat[ing]" sense of working in reproductive medicine

during this time: "we can only be overjoyed . . . to be working during a period of time when such paramount advances have been made. How thrilling it must have been to be Chaucer writing when Gutenberg invented the printing press, or to be a physicist working on the Manhattan Project!" (1983, 724). Dr. Carolyn Coulam, a professor of obstetrics and gynecology at the Mayo Clinic, similarly noted: "Within less than a quarter of a century, [new knowledge] . . . has [been] transformed . . . from the advice 'just keep trying' to the process of in vitro fertilization" (1984, 184). More developments soon followed, including the first successful live birth from an egg donation pregnancy in Australia (Lutjen et al. 1984) and the first successful live birth from a gestational surrogate pregnancy in the United States (Utian et al. 1985). The number of annual IVF-related births in the United States grew from 3,427 in 1988 to more than 20,000 by the late 1990s (Medical Research International [MRI], Society for Assisted Reproductive Technology [SART], and AFS 1990; Centers for Disease Control and Prevention [CDC], American Society for Reproductive Medicine [ASRM], and SART 2010).

AN UNORTHODOX PRACTICE? MEDICAL, LEGAL, AND RELIGIOUS RESPONSES TO AI

As a therapeutic solution for infertility, AI produced both excitement and concern. Physicians were cautious about its potential use and misuse. While some embraced both types of AI (using either husband or donor sperm), others felt that using donor sperm decidedly pushed moral, ethical, and possibly legal boundaries. In an address to the New York Obstetrical Society—later published in the *American Journal of Obstetrics and Gynecology*—Dr. Clair Folsome (1943, 923) remarked that AI with donor sperm could have "devastating [social and legal] repercussions" if it was not carried out with utmost care: "Unless . . . the marital partners are deeply earnest and understand fully the possible . . . medicolegal tangles the use of donor semen should be withheld."

The Vatican staunchly opposed any form of artificial insemination, regardless of the source of the sperm. Addressing the

Second World Congress on Fertility and Sterility, Pope Pius XII (Conte 2018, 4 and 7) observed that "involuntary conjugal sterility" could endanger marital stability but still emphasized that "it is never permissible to separate [or exclude] . . . either the procreative intention or the conjugal relationship" when treating infertility. Even though the "primary end" of marriage was the "generation and education of children," the Vatican found AI unacceptable because it separated the conjugal and procreative acts (Conte 2018, 6).

Despite caution and uncertainty within reproductive medicine and strong religious resistance from outside, many U.S. physicians offered both forms of artificial insemination (using husband and donor sperm) to their patients. Physicians often took a consequentialist perspective, emphasizing the happy outcomes of this "unorthodox" procedure (Guttmacher 1943, 591). As Dr. Alan F. Guttmacher—a preeminent obstetrician and gynecologist and advocate of reproductive rights in the twentieth century, as well as an early supporter of AID—argued, "successful artificial insemination has become one of the most satisfying of all medical experiences. It would require a petrified heart not to warm to the scene of a sterile father doting on his two children, who, according to the neighbors, resemble him very closely (1943, 591)."

In a 1947 survey of its physician members, the American Society for the Study of Sterility (ASSS; precursor to the AFS) found that 73 percent favored the practice of artificial insemination, and 62 percent had conducted AI using donor sperm or were willing to do so (Guttmacher, Haman, and MacLeod 1950). Those opposed cited numerous reasons, thinking it illegal, counter to the purpose of marriage, forbidden by religion, or generally dangerous to society. Many physicians noted the uncertain legal status of both AID and donor-conceived children, expressing concerns about illegitimacy and adultery. Given the social and legal ramifications of illegitimacy and divorce for women and children at the time, these were not just passing concerns. A 1939 editorial in *JAMA* asserted that in AI using the husband's sperm, the child was "obviously" legitimate, but a child conceived from AID "would seem to be illegitimate" even if the husband consented to the procedure (1832). However, the

American Medical Association (AMA) did not yet have a unified stance on AID. Soliciting the opinion of the AMA's Bureau of Legal Medicine, Dr. Grant S. Beardsley, an obstetrician and gynecologist in Eugene, Oregon, reported the following reply: "The offense of adultery, however defined at common law or by statute, contemplates sexual intercourse, an element of the offense which is lacking in artificial insemination" (quoted in Beardsley 1940, 97).

Many physicians were understandably concerned about the legality of AID in the absence of U.S. statutory or case law as guideposts. Additionally, the first AID court case in the Western world (*Orford v. Orford*, 1921) had ended with the Ontario Supreme Court declaring that artificial insemination using donor sperm was a form of adultery. Reading the opinion of the court, Judge J. Orde observed (1922, 22–23):

> In my judgment, the essence of the offence of adultery consists, not in the moral turpitude of the act of sexual intercourse, but in the voluntary surrender to another person of the reproductive powers or faculties . . . submission of those powers to the service or enjoyment [of anyone] other than the husband or the wife comes within the definition of "adultery." . . . In the case of the woman [committing adultery] it involves the possibility of introducing into the family of the husband a false strain of blood. . . . [T]he seed of a man other than her husband.

Compared to this early Canadian decision, the initial legal view of AID in the United States was more sympathetic. In a paper presented at the First World Congress on Fertility and Sterility (later published in *Fertility and Sterility*), Sydney B. Schatkin—then assistant corporation counsel to New York City—predicted (1954, 40 and 43): "The law's response to artificial insemination has been, and will be, perfect horror; skepticism; curiosity; and then acceptance. . . . Knowing that the law cannot be hurried, the wise doctor will continue this happiness-bestowing procedure with the conviction that the law will ultimately give its blessing."

In 1947 the New York Supreme Court ruled that a child conceived through AID with "the consent and knowledge" of the recipient woman's husband was legitimate (*Strnad v. Strnad,* 1948). Shortly afterward, a bill was introduced in the New York State Legislature "to assure the legitimacy" of donor-conceived children (Guttmacher, Haman, and MacLeod 1950, 265). Similar bills were introduced, though not enacted, in 1948–1949 in Virginia, Wisconsin, Indiana, and Minnesota (Schatkin 1954). Despite these promising steps, physicians knew they must proceed with caution: "If in a single instance the trust which the public places in those who perform donor insemination is misplaced, irreparable damage will be done to the whole medical profession" (Guttmacher 1954, 6). The legally uncertain status of AID in the United States was not over. In direct contrast to the *Strnad v. Strnad* decision, the Illinois Superior Court held that AID did constitute adultery and resulting children were illegitimate (*Doornbos v. Doornbos* 1956). Responding to this decision, the ASSS surveyed "the attitude of the membership" and released the following statement (Davis 1956, 101): "if it is in harmony with the beliefs of the couple and doctor, donor artificial insemination is a completely ethical, moral, and desirable form of medical therapy. . . . Our voice of approval should echo through the courts of law, the temples of religion, and the halls of science." Despite such explicit approval from within reproductive medicine, it would take a few more decades before state legislatures began to explicitly address (and accept) AID as a legitimate pathway to paternity.

SCIENCE FICTION OR REALITY?
THE CONTROVERSY OVER IVF

IVF invoked its own backlash in the 1970s and 1980s. Medical practitioners expressed not only excitement about the innovative therapeutic possibilities but also concern about social, legal, and ethical ramifications. DeCherney (1983, 726) cautioned: "we must take charge of the future of our field, guard against an uncontrolled technology." Some criticisms of IVF came from within reproductive medicine (e.g., how many people could actually afford to use it?), but many came from physicians in other specialties—as well as scientists, ethicists, and religious leaders.[6]

In the early 1970s, several major figures in biology, bioethics, or religion offered highly public and critical comments on the implications of IVF. In 1971, the prominent molecular biologist James Watson[7] made a formal statement on IVF to the House Committee on Science and Astronautics. Watson argued that IVF would lead to asexual reproduction and human cloning: the once "science fiction scenario" of cloning, with the potential "for misuse by an inhumane totalitarian government," was becoming a scientific reality (1971). In the same year, the physician and bioethicist Leon Kass[8] (1971, 1174 and 1178) published an article in the *New England Journal of Medicine*, questioning whether IVF constituted "unethical experiments on the unborn" and was "exploit[ing] . . . the desires of a childless couple." An anonymous *JAMA* editorial on "genetic engineering in man" in the following year concluded: "the time seems clearly at hand to declare a moratorium on experiments that would attempt to implant an in vitro conceptus into a woman's womb" ("Genetic Engineering in Man" 1972). The next two *JAMA* issues featured essays by Paul Ramsey (1972a and 1972b), a Princeton University professor of religion and medical ethics, describing IVF as "unethical medical experimentation" that should be "subject to absolute moral prohibition" (1972a, 1346).

The Roman Catholic Church also heavily criticized IVF, as an extension of its earlier stance on AI. In 1987 the Congregation for the Doctrine of the Faith—an office of the Vatican responsible for ""promot[ing] and safeguard[ing] doctrine regarding faith and morals throughout the Catholic world" (Holy See 2018)—published "Instruction on Respect for Human Life in its Origins and on the Dignity of Procreation: Replies to Certain Questions of the Day." Noting the "great urgency" required to clarify a Catholic position, the document described both IVF and AI as undermining marital unity, offending the dignity of spouses, and violating the rights of children to be both conceived and born within the confines of marriage. It also emphasized the need to respect "the human being . . . from the very first instant of his existence" (Congregation for the Doctrine of the Faith 1987).

Similar to AI, IVF created substantial legal uncertainty. However, concerns about IVF focused primarily on the legal and ethical status of embryos and gametes, rather than on parentage and family issues. In 1973, the U.S. Department of Health, Education, and Welfare (HEW)—precursor to the Department of Health and Human Services—required that any research seeking federal funding must first be reviewed by an ethics board. The first submitted proposal led to the creation of the HEW Ethics Advisory Board and a series of public hearings in 1978–1979 (Quigley and Andrews 1984). The subsequent HEW report supported continuing IVF research (Ethics Advisory Board 1979), but by 1980 the board had "ceased to exist," creating a de facto moratorium on federally funded IVF research (Quigley and Andrews 1984, 349). During that same period, a president's commission was created to address ethics in medicine and in biomedical and behavioral research (Capron 1983). The commission was instructed to finish its work by December 1982 (Capron 1983). From 1980 to 1982, it released nine reports on various ethical issues in biomedicine and medical research. None addressed IVF. In the early 1990s, the AFS and the American College of Obstetricians and Gynecologists provided seed funding for an ethics board in the interest of having an independent advisory board (Cohen 1996). This developed into the National Advisory Board on Ethics in Reproduction, an external, interdisciplinary body formed in 1991 to discuss ethical and policy issues related to reproductive technologies. However, this was ultimately a private-sector alternative to fill the decade-long vacuum of a much-needed national forum.

The lack of federal guidance on IVF research and therapy during the 1970s and 1980s was a huge loss, especially in the tumultuous climate of reproductive politics after the U.S. Supreme Court decision in *Roe v. Wade* (1973). In *Roe*, the Supreme Court considered abortion as falling within the constitutional right to privacy, consistent with prior decisions on contraception (Weitz 2009). The Court also granted significant power to physicians to use their expert discretion in deciding whether abortion was necessary for a patient. Political backlash against *Roe* came in the form of a series of state-level restrictions against research using aborted fetuses or involving pregnant women who intended to terminate their pregnancies or might be coerced into doing so. Though not explicitly anticipating IVF, many statutes defined 'fetus' broadly to refer to any products of conception and thus had implications for IVF (Quigley and Andrews 1984). Some states passed laws to specifically restrict or monitor IVF. In 1979, an Illinois statute addressing abortion was amended to include IVF. Physicians who manipulated reproductive cells in vitro were deemed to have "care and custody" of the cells as future children and could therefore be accused of endangering their life or health under a child welfare statute from the late nineteenth century (Quigley and Andrews 1984, 349). A 1986 act in Louisiana defined IVF-created embryos as 'juridical persons' with certain rights and interests that needed protection. While the Louisiana law had rather minimal impact on IVF, seeming to serve a mostly symbolic function (at the time), the Illinois law decidedly had a temporary chilling effect: physicians were "unwilling to [conduct IVF procedures] under the threat of such liability" (Simon 1991, 138). After challenges by prospective IVF patients and their physicians, the Illinois statute was amended to remove the language addressing IVF procedures. However, the Louisiana law still stands—an issue I address more fully in chapter 6.

Frustrated with the lack of external leadership and the de facto moratorium on IVF research, the AFS published its own ethical statement on IVF (AFS 1984). The ad hoc committee that wrote the statement, chaired by Dr. Howard Jones, later became the AFS Committee on Ethics. This new committee was tasked with formulating reports and position statements to guide practitioners as they reckoned with the moral, legal, and social implications of their work. To bolster the ethical case for assisted reproduction, the AFS also needed support outside of reproductive medicine. The first committee members provided expertise from different social worlds: they included attorneys, developmental and reproductive biologists, ethicists, obstetricians and gynecologists, an endocrinologist and andrologist, and a moral theologian (AFS Committee on Ethics 1986). Even with such a diverse membership, the first committee report unanimously concluded: "basic IVF is ethically acceptable" (33S).

In terms of immediate ethical concerns, the committee also needed to address the status of the pre-embryo. This term referred to a period in embryonic development occurring after fertilization but prior to the appearance of the 'primitive streak.' This refers to a faint streak that is the precursor to the spinal cord, identifying the earliest formation of an embryo during the fourteen-day period directly after fertilization (Wilson 1914). During IVF procedures, this was the period when physicians transferred embryos back into the recipient woman's uterus. Other organizations and experts, such as members of the HEW Ethics Advisory Board, had signaled the symbolic importance of this period, raising concerns about the moral and legal status of the pre-embryo (Ethics Advisory Board 1979). AFS members editorialized on this issue in *Fertility and Sterility* (Coulam 1984; Gleicher 1984; H. Jones 1982, 1989, and 1990). Most repeated the current scientific knowledge: fertilization was a process, not a singular event. There were no formal biological markers of such concepts as 'ensoulment' or 'personhood.' Embryonic losses (i.e., early pregnancy loss during the embryonic phase of gestation) frequently occurred in natural reproduction, perhaps at a greater rate than during IVF procedures. Reproductive cells were alive (how could they be otherwise?) and considered human in nature. However, although some might be potential people, medically, socially, or legally they should not be considered full-fledged people. The status of the pre-embryo was particularly salient in the aftermath of *Roe v. Wade* (1973). Physicians working in reproductive medicine could use *Roe* to assert that interventions in early pregnancy, such as IVF, were a private matter between the woman and her doctor. At the same time, many such physicians aimed to distance their work from abortion politics, asserting that they were doing quite the opposite from abortion: creating wanted pregnancies for the desperately, hopelessly infertile.

In sum, both AI and IVF prompted excitement as well as concern from medical, legal, and religious sources. However, the central concerns about the two techniques focused on distinct issues. Concerns about AI, and specifically the use of donor sperm, highlighted that the procedure was a potential threat to the legal and social stability of the traditional, heteropatriarchal institutions of marriage and family, raising the specters of adultery and illegitimacy by introducing another man into biological reproduction. Who was the "real" father of a donor-conceived child? Were these techniques legal? Moral? In the best interests of the future child and family unit? In contrast, concerns about IVF intermingled with abortion politics in the post-*Roe* era, steering the discussion more toward concerns about the sanctity of human life and the notions of personhood and humanness. Was an embryo alive? Was it a person? Was IVF a slippery slope to cloning and asexual reproduction? How many embryo-lives would be lost during IVF research and therapy? These distinct frames—of politics of family versus politics of life—set the stage for quite different conversations about the meanings of AI and IVF as modes of family building. In the next section I look more specifically at conversations within reproductive medicine. Against the historical and cultural backdrop that I have just described, how did physicians (and a few other prominently featured outside experts and commentators) make sense of the reproductive work they were doing? (How) Did they think about the implications of using donor gametes for paternity and maternity?

Making Sense of Gamete Donation

RESTORING (THE FAÇADE OF) BIOPATERNITY

Physicians in reproductive medicine viewed AID's main social problem as its creating "split paternity," with "one biologic father and a different assumed father" (Guttmacher, Haman, and MacLeod 1950, 264). By introducing two possible fathers into the picture, AID appeared akin to adultery. It might destroy marriages that were already unstable because of the stress of infertility and childlessness. Given AID's early uncertain legal status, physicians were also concerned about their role and liability in offering AID therapy. Dr. Sophia Kleegman[9]—a gynecologist, birth control advocate, and infertility expert—cautioned that physicians might be held liable on two possible grounds (1954, 9): "first, as committing adultery by introduction of semen not the husband's [sic] into the wife; and second, as conspiracy to commit adultery since the physician was the go-between in the introduction of semen from the donor." Others argued that AID was not technically adultery but still implied it. In a symposium on AID in *Fertility and Sterility*, Fowler Harper, a professor at Yale University's law school, noted (quoted in Buxton 1958, 375): "Adultery implies the penetration of a man's penis into the genital tract of a woman, one of the parties being married to a third person. This does not happen in A.I.D. But the birth of issue to a married woman by a man other than her husband implies adultery. This does happen in A.I.D. A whole host of legal complexities arise [sic] from these anomalies."

Some physicians expressed the fear that a husband would reject a nonbiological child. If the marriage should dissolve, he might not pay child support, or he might seek to disinherit the child, stating his own sterility as evidence of the child's illegitimacy (Seashore 1938; Seymour and Koerner 1936; Shields 1950). Drs. Frances Seymour and Alfred Koerner (1936, 1532) described how they carefully guarded against this potential problem by having the husband and the wife sign a consent form, "sworn to before a notary," and place their fingerprints "next to their respective signatures." The consent forms "signed in duplicate, notarized and witnessed," were then "separated and placed respectively in the vaults of separate banks and forgotten unless legal complications should arise." Having the couple undergo such a consent process served to both "legitimize the child" and act "as a mental binder on the husband . . . he knows that he can never deny having authorized the creation of his wife's child."

Other physicians worried that a wife, in her willingness to push the boundaries of social conventions, would end up shunned by the community, extended family, or eventually the donor-conceived child. Remarking on the "social propriety" of donor insemination, Dr. Folsome (1943, 924) cautioned: "the woman, made pregnant by . . . donor semen, who even whispers out of turn, on a single occasion, becomes a medical curiosity . . . shunned by her relatives and perhaps unfortunately her own child. . . . The so-called veneer of civilized culture is thin, none the less it is of an oppressive nature to the woman willing to overstep the bounds of her environmental social mores and wedlock in her real desire to have a child of her own."

Even given these concerns, many physicians found AID to be a highly useful therapy for infertile patients and therefore aimed to normalize the procedure. One strategy was to compare AID to adoption, which provided a ready framework for a nonbiological relationship between parent and child. Adoption was also ethically palatable as a more socially accepted, if marginalized, mode of family building. In a 1957 article in *Fertility and Sterility*, Dr. Fred A. Simmons—a physician at Harvard Medical School and Massachusetts General Hospital—observed the use of the adoption analogy among his colleagues (1957, 548): "Ethnologically, adoption is defined as the receiving into the clan or tribe of one from outside, and treating him as one of the same blood. The role of the husband in therapeutic insemination is simply that." However, this comparison was limited because adoption acknowledged biological discontinuity in the father-child relationship, a characteristic presumed to create more tenuous ties than kinship based on biology (Wegar 1998). Another limitation of the adoption analogy was that some physicians felt that AID was superior to adoption. AID allowed husbands to be more involved by going through the experience of pregnancy and birth with their wives. This could create a greater sense of connection to the child and stabilize the infertile husband's place within the family. He could more readily "consider the child his": "he requests in writing that the doctor make it possible for his wife to have a child by insemination and by the time the child arrives, the husband says to himself: 'I asked for this child and it is mine.' He feels that he has helped to make his marriage complete, which he was unable to do before. He feels that he has made it possible for his wife to experience the pleasures of normal pregnancy and he, in fact, has shared the pleasures and the problems of the ensuing 280 days of gestation" (Simmons 1957, 548).

If the infertile husband was capable of producing any sperm at all, a few physicians recommended that his semen be mixed with that of the donor "to introduce the element of uncertainty" (Shields 1950, 275) and suggest that the child might in fact be his biological offspring.[10] One such case, reported by Dr. Frances Shields in a 1950 article in *Fertility and Sterility*, involved a woman whose husband had azoospermia (the absence of sperm in his seminal fluid). The couple conceived a child using donor sperm, but the wife never sought a second pregnancy by this method: "her husband was convinced by some miracle that [the first donor-conceived child] was his child. She knew if she had more inseminations and became pregnant [again] he would realize that neither baby was his. She had decided, and I believe wisely, not to disturb his conviction that he *was* a [biological] father" (Shields 1950, 279).

One can see evidence of the great lengths that some physicians went to in the interest of preserving the natural and (hetero)sexual elements of conjugal reproduction even while using donor sperm. For instance, in an article in the *American Journal of Surgery*, a Dr. C. Travers Stepita of New York (1933, 450) described a procedure whereby a husband with azoospermia would be catheterized and injected with "alien" (i.e., donor) sperm, followed by normal coitus in the hope of creating an "opportunity for impregnation . . . in a perfectly natural and physiologic manner." Although this method did not catch on widely, many other physicians did recommend that couples have intercourse the night of the insemination procedure "to give the [donor] sperm a boost" and to provide the husband with "a sense of helpful participation" in conception (Kleegman 1954, 21).

Most importantly, AID could preserve the outward façade of biological paternity, thereby restoring the social continuity of the father-child relationship and allowing the husband to assume his rightful role: "In the eyes of the community the couple are Mr. and

Mrs. X with their child or children, rather than Mr. and Mrs. X with their 'adopted' child. . . . The husband is able to take his place in the community as the normal head of a normal family" (Simmons 1957, 548–549). While some physicians still urged husbands to legally adopt donor-conceived children, others argued that this might disturb the delicate façade of biological paternity, assumed to be of utmost importance in both salvaging the husband's masculinity and creating a so-called normal family.

IT'S ALL UNDER (MEDICAL) CONTROL

Physicians were well aware of the need to contain and control AID as a potentially deviant medical practice. Medical social control refers to the means by which medicine as an institution, and medical practitioners as individuals, seek to minimize, eliminate, or normalize deviance (Conrad 1992). In an interesting twist, gamete donation represents a case in which the deviant behavior originated within medicine. Thus, social control was needed both to contain potential sociolegal harms and to maintain the professional reputation of reproductive medicine. Dr. Abner I. Weisman—a physician at the Evangelical Deaconess Hospital in Brooklyn—(1942, 144) noted solemnly: "[the physician] has taken upon himself not only the scientific treatment but also the legal 'guardianship' of a family that has placed in him the opportunity of creating very life itself." Similarly, Guttmacher (quoted in Buxton 1958, 370) observed: "in the ethical sense, whenever a physician performs donor insemination he is substituting for The Creator. This is no mean responsibility."

Patient gatekeeping by physicians offered one crucial method of control over AID. Such gatekeeping was understood as normal and expected under the dominant paradigm of physician paternalism and the traditional medical model of infertility treatment during this period (Braverman 2010; Daniels and Golden 2004). Most physicians treated only infertile married couples, containing the uses of AID to a morally 'acceptable' patient population.[11] Physicians also stressed their responsibility to assess the suitability of the prospective parents. Beardsley (1940, 95) observed that the requesting couple "should be of a high moral and intellectual type, and financially able to give the child the educational advantages demanded of their social station." He further reported that the "Seymour group" (headed by Dr. Frances Seymour) required "a minimum I.Q. of 120 in all receptive mothers" as well as a guarantee that the prospective parents would provide for the child's education. While some physicians clearly had an interest in promoting positive eugenics through the selective use of donor insemination (for a lengthier discussion of this, see Daniels and Golden 2004; see also Weisman 1942), others seemed more intent on minimizing sociolegal disruptions and physician liability. Dr. Sophia Kleegman (1954, 28) urged: "choice of couple must be based on a sound and stable marriage, a complete emotional acceptance of and preference for this procedure by both husband and wife, and their true love of children." Dr. Louis Portnoy, a physician affiliated with the Margaret Sanger Research Bureau in New York, similarly described his clinical criteria in an article in *Fertility and Sterility*: "intelligence, understanding of what they are about to undertake, emotional equipment for parenthood, the stability of their marriage, and the sincerity of their desire for a child by this method" (1956, 329).

Physicians also maintained tight control over donor selection. Weisman (1942, 142) reported that "the couple should be informed at the very first that the selection of a donor must be entirely left to the judgment of the physician." To preserve the façade of biological paternity, physicians aimed to select a donor who at least matched the husband's physical appearance, racial identity, and blood type. They also considered such factors as religion and so-called temperament of the husband. Donors needed to be in good health and have both an upstanding character and a clean family medical history. Medical students or residents at a local hospital provided a ready and a renewable donor source. In an article in *JAMA*, Guttmacher reported purchasing "semen specimens . . . from medical students or [hospital] staff members for $5 each" (1942, 443)—a practice that seemed both suitable and convenient to many physicians. These men were trusted to be available on short notice as well as be less likely to transmit infections than the "general warp and woof of our society" (Kleegman 1954, 27). Guttmacher later noted (1943, 589) that the men in this donor pool "are of such a type [intellectually and physically] that I truthfully feel the child to be conceived is fortunate to have so superior a father."

However, some physicians cautioned against using younger, unmarried medical students who might be "prone to affliction by some mental disease": a stable family man who had proven his own fertility was likely a wiser choice (Weisman 1942, 143). Using friends or male relatives was almost unanimously considered problematic for several reasons (Beardsley 1940; Kleegman 1954; Seashore 1938; Weisman 1942). The wife, technically carrying the biological child of another man, might start to think about the known donor or even transfer her affections to the man whose semen had impregnated her, leading to an "estrangement of [her] affections" from her husband (Seashore 1938, 643). The known donor might undermine the nuclear family unit by attempting to establish his own paternity (thereby nullifying the husband's) and seeking custody of the child. In the interest of family harmony, physicians stressed that the donor should "remain the *forgotten man*" (Beardsley 1940, 96)—fading into the background after the AI procedure.

Physicians considered anonymity and secrecy to be essential for the successful practice of AID. Sperm donors and recipient couples were kept anonymous from one another within hospitals and clinics. Physicians also urged couples to keep the details of conception secret from friends and family members. Some physicians who oversaw the insemination procedure referred couples to a different practitioner for pregnancy care and delivery. Not knowing the full history of conception, the second physician would not even think to ask if the husband was the biological father and would "fill out the birth certificate naming husband and wife as the parents of the child" (Kleegman 1954, 11). Such a "white lie" was "perfectly justified" (Shields 1950, 278) to assist the husband and wife in forgetting that AID had even happened and move ahead as a family. Decades after these physician discussions, the medical anthropologist Gay Becker (2000 and 2002) showed that whether to tell sperm donor–conceived children about the facts of their conception was still an "unresolved" (2002) issue among U.S. couples because of the cultural privileging of biological parenthood and the threat of male infertility to heteromasculinity.

A MORE NATURAL AND NORMAL TECHNOLOGY

Compared to the concerning "split paternity" in AID, women using egg donation still retained some biological connection to their child. Was it such a major issue to replace only half of women's biological contribution? Because egg donation preserved the gestational relationship, it also did not overtly undermine the legal presumption of maternity. And, arguably, pregnancy has been considered more culturally and socially important to maternity than genes. Genes are less publicly visible and do not always translate in expected ways from parent to child. However, pregnancy is highly visible and central to the rituals and norms of expectant motherhood (Teman 2010; Rothman 1989). Both physicians and prominent outside experts commenting on egg donation seemed to start from these premises. They drew comparisons between egg donation and its immediately relevant alternatives, adoption and traditional surrogacy (gestational surrogacy would come later), to argue that egg donation was a more natural mode of family building. They focused on the promise of IVF-based therapies for treating patients that they viewed as hopelessly or desperately infertile, framing egg donation as a highly moral medical solution to end human suffering. And because by this point AID had been in practice for several decades, they likened egg donation to the female variant of AID—just switch the gender of the donor, recipient, and spouse.

As an ardent promoter and defender of IVF in the 1970s, Dr. Howard Jones (1983, 2182) also staunchly defended egg donation as a treatment option for "desperate couples" seeking parenthood. In an early commentary in *JAMA*, Jones (1983) argued that of all the options available to infertile women at the time, egg donation was both more natural and less controversial than adoption and surrogacy. Likening the practice to a superior type of "intrauterine adoption," he noted (1983, 2183): "child adoption is considered highly ethical in most segments of society . . . [and] while there is a big difference between a child and a conceptus . . . it can even be argued that parental instincts may be increased by intrauterine adoption rather than later adoption." In the same *JAMA* issue, LeRoy Walters (director of the Kennedy Institute's Center for Bioethics at Georgetown University and later a member of the first AFS Ethics Committee) noted (1983, 2184): "[egg donation] most closely approximates the usual process of human reproduction. Both members of the couple are directly involved in the pregnancy, the man through providing semen and the woman through carrying the pregnancy . . . and giving birth. . . . [Therefore] preimplantation adoption should be less disruptive to the family unit [than surrogacy]." Over a decade later, Drs. David Barad and Brian Cohen (medical directors of an early egg donor program at Montefiore Medical Center in New York) echoed these sentiments, arguing that they were simply giving nature a bit of help in the beginning (1996, 16, 27):

> There seems to be greater justice in oocyte donation than in surrogacy . . . those who benefit from the procedure bear the risks of pregnancy. Oocyte donation also seems more natural, in that the mother who gives birth will raise the child. . . .
>
> Even the most sophisticated of technologies does not "make" a baby. . . . [A surgeon] uses suture to attach tissues atraumatically and reconstruct natural relationships. . . . Assisted reproductive technology allows physicians to facilitate reproduction in much the same way. . . . [B]ring[ing] the components of reproduction into contact with each other. If we do our job well, nature will take its course.

Thus, egg donation was frequently framed as "more natural" than other assisted and collaborative reproductive options, approximating "the usual process" of reproduction. However, most commentators and physicians did not directly address the fact that maternal genetics were replaced with donor genetics. Those who did downplayed the significance of women's genetic connection. The genetic loss was considered less important than what egg donation could do for the desperately infertile woman. Responding to the Roman Catholic position against IVF and arguing for the "ethical acceptab[ility]" of donor gametes, the AFS Committee on Ethics stated in a report (1988, 2S): "As an alternative to childbearing with conjugal gametes . . . the principle of using heterologous [donor] gametes presents a justifiable relaxation of unity between the genetic and gestational components of procreation." Notably, this "relaxation of unity" applied only to donor eggs that were gestated by the intended mother, not gestational surrogacy in which another woman gestated the embryo for the intended parents. Many physicians shared this sentiment, expressing the greater importance of gestational over genetic maternity. For instance, Drs. Barad and Cohen (1996, 26) asserted that "the gestational mother is not a passive vessel [in egg donation], but an active force in the creation of new life. Motherhood brings much more than genetics to reproduction." Reflecting on the "historical evolution" of U.S. egg donation, Dr. John Buster (director of the Department of Obstetrics and Gynecology at Baylor College of Medicine) observed (1998,7): "Even though women will prefer to bear children with their own genetic characteristics, for many there is no better choice [than egg donation]."

If egg donation was considered more natural than other family-building modes, it was also seen as not wildly different from AID. Indeed, by the time egg donation was introduced in the early 1980s, AID had been regularly used in medical practice for over half a century and had been a medically recognized treatment for nearly a century. AID offered an intuitive, preexisting model that could help neutralize concerns. Reporting in a *JAMA* article on the first clinical trial in the United States using nonsurgical ovum transfer methods, Dr. Maria Bustillo and colleagues (1984, 1173) stated matter-of-factly: "As a legal issue, the process of ovum transfer, although more [medically] complicated, is in concept analogous to artificial insemination by donor, which is a well-established infertility therapy." In the same issue of *JAMA*, Grace Ganz Blumberg, a law professor at the University of California, Los Angeles, made a similar case that AID offered a clear precedent for deciding in favor of the "uterine mother": "ovum transfer merely reverses the gender roles of AID. . . . [T]he logic of AID statutes requires that the . . . husband be treated as the child's father. . . . [Therefore] the recipient uterine mother . . . should treated as the legal mother" (1984, 1180). In a more official capacity, the 1993 "Guidelines for Oocyte Donation," written by the AFS's Ad Hoc Committee of the Society for Assisted Reproductive Technology (precursor to SART), described donated oocytes as "medically analogous" to donated sperm, the latter of which "has been medically recognized as a treatment for otherwise uncorrectable male infertility for a hundred years" (1993, 5S). Intriguingly, although many medical practitioners and nonmedical experts compared egg donation with AID to normalize the former, both techniques were consistently designated as "ethically acceptable" but "controversial" by the AFS Committee on Ethics throughout the 1980s and 1990s (1986, 1988, 1990, and 1994).

SUSPICION AND CONCERN

One notable difference between egg donation and sperm donation was that physicians paid substantially more attention to the motivations and experiences of egg donors relative to sperm donors. Physicians expressed both suspicion and concern about potential egg donors. Logistically, eggs are scarcer and more difficult to retrieve from the human body than sperm. Extracting them requires more invasive procedures, especially when considering early IVF and the laparoscopic techniques that physicians used. Yet some discussions also reflected assumptions that women were more emotionally invested in their eggs as future potential children than men were in their sperm (Almeling 2011; Johnson 2017a) or that women would seek to donate for the 'wrong' reasons. Egg donation came with its own set of medical and social risks that centered more directly on the donor, in direct contrast to the view that sperm donors should become the "forgotten man" in AID (Beardsley 1940, 96).

Early on, practitioners used both in vivo (in the body) fertilization and in vitro (in glass) fertilization (i.e., IVF) methods for egg donation (Bustillo et al. 1984; Rosenwaks 1987). For in vivo cases, egg donors underwent artificial insemination using the intended sperm, typically from the egg recipient's husband. Fertilization and early pre-embryonic development happened inside the donor's body. This was followed by nonsurgical uterine lavage to flush out the pre-embryo, which was then transferred to the recipient woman's body for implantation and gestation. In IVF cases, physicians surgically retrieved eggs from the donor's body,[12] fertilized these in vitro using the intended sperm, and then transferred the pre-embryo to the recipient woman's body for implantation and gestation. The donor's body was more central in the case of the in vivo and uterine lavage method, creating more medical and social risks. Donors might acquire a pelvic infection, be exposed to a sexually transmitted infection, or have an ectopic pregnancy—potentially damaging their own fertility in the process of donating (Bustillo et al. 1983; H. Jones 1983; AFS Committee on Ethics 1986). Physicians also questioned egg donors' abilities to comply with medical orders, as well as their overall trustworthiness and motives for undergoing the procedure. If a donor did not abstain from intercourse during the proper window of time, she could have sperm from her sexual partner in her reproductive tract, which could mingle with the intended sperm from the insemination procedure and introduce uncertainty about biological paternity (Blumberg 1984; Bustillo et al. 1983; Jones H. 1983). Like AID, the in vivo method also raised the specter of sexual intimacy and adultery, because the egg donor was directly inseminated with the recipient's husband's sperm. For a brief period, their united gametes were housed inside of her body, violating conjugal exclusivity. On the more extreme end, some commenters envisioned uterine "holdup[s]" (Blumberg 1984, 1180), with a donor accidentally or intentionally refusing lavage after fertilization and thus retaining the pregnancy, holding the embryo for ransom from a wealthy, infertile couple. Given the greater physical and social risks involved with the in vivo fertilization and lavage approach for egg donation, the AFS Committee on Ethics (1986, 48S) noted "serious reservations . . . about this method in its current state." Work on the in vivo and lavage approach was discontinued in the United States by 1987 (Buster 1998; Sauer and Kavic 2006). However, the IVF method for egg donation was not without its own set of risks. Many of these were connected to the source of donated oocytes.

OOCYTES WANTED

Oocyte supply was a consistent problem from the beginning. Practitioners identified four potential sources: IVF patients with excess eggs; tubal ligation patients; designated donors, such as friends or female family members; and volunteer (paid) donors from the broader community. Initially women in the first two groups were more commonly used because they were already undergoing laparoscopic procedures. Practitioners were wary of using healthy women who had no other reason to have surgery. This would change later, with the introduction of transvaginal ultrasound-guided aspiration (Dellenbach et al. 1985)—a much less invasive method of retrieving oocytes compared to the original laparoscopic methods used (which involved surgical retrieval through a small incision in the abdomen, performed under general anesthesia). Additionally, with advancements in embryo cryopreservation, many IVF patients began freezing their excess embryos rather than donating them (Trounson 1986). Physicians also began relying less on IVF patients as donors amid growing concerns that "disputes over . . . disclosure, ownership, and custody" would be more likely to happen if the patient had not first successfully formed her own family (Sauer and Paulson 1992, 17). Using patients' eggs fell further out of favor after a 1992 scandal involving clinical misuse of cryopreserved embryos (J. Roberts 1995; Sauer and Kavic 2006). Three prominent physicians in U.S. reproductive medicine, who were also faculty members at the University of California, Irvine, were accused of misappropriating patients' excess embryos—using the embryos for other patients without permission and even selling some embryos to research laboratories (Roberts 1995). There were nearly 140 cases in which eggs or embryos "disappeared [from the university-based fertility clinic] . . . and were then distributed to other women, used for research or lost" (B. Jones 2009). In 2009, the university finally settled with the plaintiffs and brought the litigation to an end.

All these issues created greater demand for alternative donor sources. Sisters of infertile women offered an intuitive and readily available option. In contrast to the taboo against using male relatives in AID, sister-to-sister egg donation was generally considered culturally acceptable (Sauer et al. 1988; Lessor 1993). Surveying couples undergoing either AID or egg donation treatment, Dr. Mark Sauer and colleagues (1988, 722) found a striking difference in views about sibling donors: "[most egg donation patients] had not only considered [their sister] . . . but had already approached her. . . . 61% had secured such an agreement. . . . On the contrary, few (11%) couples undergoing AID preferred using a brother as their donor, and none had asked one to participate." But some practitioners expressed concern that sisters might feel compelled to donate eggs to family members instead of doing so of their own volition (Klein, Sewall, and Soules 1996; Barad and Cohen 1996). For instance, in discussing the process for screening a "known [egg] donor," Dr. Nancy Klein and colleagues at the University of Washington Medical Center noted that "particular attention is paid to psychosocial issues and motivation . . . with an effort to identify possible coercion" (1996, 9). To avoid the potential for such coercion, some fertility clinics began to experiment with volunteer donors by recruiting women from the general public to serve as compensated donors. Using this last source of oocytes is now standard practice in contemporary U.S. egg donation (Almeling 2011; Johnson 2017a and 2017b).

As programs shifted to using volunteer, compensated donors, physicians and ethicists alike had reservations about who would come forward to donate. Some of their suspicion was connected to donor compensation, which dramatically increased during the 1990s as U.S. egg donation was transformed into a medical market quite different from that for sperm donation (Almeling 2011; Johnson 2017b; Spar 2006). Other misgivings arose from a distinctively gendered discomfort with egg donation: what type of woman would voluntarily give away her eggs? Clinical donation programs began implementing more stringent gatekeeping of potential donors (Johnson 2017a). While some measures (e.g., screening for sexually transmitted infections) were medically necessary, others reflected cultural and professional anxieties. Describing their volunteer donor recruitment in an article in *Fertility and Sterility*, Dr. Elizabeth Kennard and colleagues at the Cleveland Clinic Foundation noted that "the only absolute requirements" for donors were "general good health, age 18 through 35, and normal menstrual cycles" (1989, 656). However, their article further revealed that donor recruitment actually involved a rigorous medical and psychological screening process, including getting consent from the donor's husband if she was married; conducting a psychological interview to assess her motivations, expectations, and support from family members or friends regarding the donation; a thorough history of emotional trauma and intimate relationships; and a final interview with a bioethicist to assess informed consent. The authors explicitly excluded women who reported any history of "reproductive trauma" (658), which included such experiences as having a nonmarital pregnancy, an abortion, or a partner who refused to have children. They also excluded women with any history of "family trauma" or a "disrupted family," (658) such as divorce, the death of a parent, or a family member who abused drugs or alcohol. And they excluded any women who were primarily motivated by "financial gain" (658). This level of screening and exclusion criteria for egg donation was a far cry from the early days of sperm donation, when physicians often relied on healthy and willing medical students as donors.

Physicians also raised the concern that women might be using egg donation as a way to 'repent' for past reproductive actions like abortion or lost reproductive opportunities. These concerns reflected cultural beliefs that women have a strong, innate drive to bear children and would have a difficult time separating their own reproductive desires from the eggs they planned to donate. As noted above, Drs. Kennard and colleagues (1989, 658) specifically singled out any reports of "family trauma" or "reproductive trauma" as factors "that could have influenced [women's] decision to volunteer for oocyte donation"—framing egg donation as a potentially deviant act by women with nonnormative reproductive histories. When Drs. Barad and Cohen (1996, 16) found that donors in their program had a higher rate of past voluntary abortion than the general population, they speculated: "oocyte donation was [likely] an act of contrition for them. Or it may be that they placed less value on the products of their reproductive processes than women who did not choose to be donors. More than half of our donors have been unmarried and many of them do not plan to have children of their own. Oocyte donation may allow these women to fulfill their own urge to reproduce." In a notable edited volume titled *Principles of Oocyte and Embryo Donation*, Dr. Marsha Gorrill, a professor of obstetrics, gynecology, and reproductive endocrinology at Oregon Health Sciences University, advised care in exploring both "short-term and long-term psychological effects of egg donation" prior to accepting a donor:

> It is important to determine the donor's ability to emotionally separate the act of donating her eggs from the child that might be conceived. . . . Many donors have children and value motherhood and they may have a friend or family member who has experienced infertility. Some egg donors do not plan to have children, and egg donation may allow them to fulfill their own urge to reproduce. A desire to atone for previous reproductive losses may be a factor in deciding to participate as an egg donor for some women with a history of previous elective termination of pregnancy (1998, 44–45).

The psychologist Andrea Mechanick Braverman strongly advocated for psychological investigation in gamete donation. She also advised egg donation programs to develop clear protocols and involve mental health professionals:

> The ovum donor needs to be fully capable and free from any coercion. . . . [T]he prevalence of sexual abuse and trauma among [U.S.] women adds another consideration about . . . long-term sequelae of performing an invasive procedure . . . [We must] evaluate the psychological issues involved . . . rather than . . . assume there are none because little psychological research and evaluation have been done on sperm donors.
>
> [Ovum] donors need to be evaluated for both psychopathology and for their ability to anticipate the psychological unknowns and stresses in going through the donor cycle. For example, does the donor understand and accept the boundaries of her role? (Braverman and the Ovum Donor Task Force of the Psychological Special Interests Group of the American Fertility Society 1993, 1219–1220)

Not all practitioners felt concern about egg donors' mental state or ability to let go of their eggs. The medical sociologist Roberta Lessor and colleagues from the University of California, Irvine Medical Center (1993, 67) reported that their donors were "maternal" but not in a way that might threaten the recipient's maternity: "[our donors are] socially conventional, outgoing, and free from psychopathology. . . . They took pride in their maternal capacities. Those who had given birth indicated . . . [it was] a high point of their lives . . . they would like to make possible for a recipient." Others were openly critical of the extensive screening measures used for egg donors. Reflecting on early egg donation days in the United States, Dr. Mark Sauer (1996, 1149) observed: "The double standard was obviously sexist, yet could not be dismissed. To appease critics [of egg donation] certain 'safeguards' were invoked to address the myriad of newly identified concerns. Psychologists were introduced into the formal screening process of donors and recipients. Lawyers and hospital administrators were consulted. . . . As a result, oocyte donation has grown to become complicated and expensive."

Another clear departure from AID was in regard to the expectations for anonymity and secrecy. Anonymity and confidentiality about the terms of conception were standard practice and relatively easy to institute when donor eggs primarily came from other IVF patients. Practitioners were concerned that an infertility patient's donation might result in pregnancy for another woman, but her own cycle might be unsuccessful, causing a dispute over any resulting child. But anonymity was clearly impossible when couples used a designated donor such as a sister or friend. Thus, while the AFS generally considered anonymity to be desirable in gamete donation it was not always practical in egg donation specifically. Beyond practicalities, there was simply not the same emphasis on secrecy in egg donation—even though secrecy was so essential to AID. With the common early use of known egg donors, there was little that professional medicine could do to closely guard the secrets of donor egg conception. But another reason that secrecy was less salient to egg donation is in the inherent asymmetry in the male and female reproductive roles. Men's only biological paternal connection was fully severed by sperm donation, but egg donation did not wholly undermine biological maternity. Unlike the delicate façade of biological paternity in AID—which was maintained by careful secrecy, anonymity, and physician control—biological maternity via pregnancy was still a publicly visible fact, even for women using donor eggs. Braverman pointed to this apparent "double standard" in gamete donation, noting that prior studies emphasized the need for anonymity in AID to "protect the self-esteem of the male" as well as the father-child relationship, but "the ovum donor recipient has the gestational contribution to the pregnancy" (Braverman and the Ovum Donor Task Force of the Psychological Special Interests Group of the American Fertility Society 1993, 1219). Braverman asked: "does [gestation] allay our fears about the potentially negative impact of using a donor?" The overwhelming sentiment within reproductive medicine suggested that the answer was yes. The social visibility and legal emphasis on pregnancy and birth seemed to salvage biological maternity, even if a woman used donor eggs.

The different eras when sperm and egg donation first emerged and gained momentum as medical therapies contributed to differences in how they were practiced and interpreted. AID emerged when the eugenics movement was at its height in the United States and physician paternalism was the dominant mode of medical practice. IVF and egg donation came on the heels of women's liberation and gains in reproductive rights, including access to contraception and abortion. The women's health and patient rights movements of the 1970s spurred new philosophies in doctor-patient interactions, emphasizing patient-centered care and informed consent as a corrective to physician paternalism. Charis Thompson (2005) has noted other transformations specific to reproductive medicine, where patient gatekeeping practices shifted from an initial litmus test of what was considered to be in the 'best interests of the child' to 'reproductive choice and privacy.' This shift is seen in the notable absence of gatekeeping for egg donation patients compared to strict physician control over patient selection for AID. AID tested the cultural waters first and was met with significant early backlash, as it was viewed as threatening to marriage and family life. IVF stirred its own set of controversies in the post-*Roe* political landscape, provoking concerns about the moral and legal status of the pre-embryo. Yet only a few years later, in the early 1980s, practitioners discussed egg donation as a relatively normal and natural technique used in helping infertile women have babies, strategically drawing comparisons to adoption, traditional surrogacy, and AID in the process.

In a cultural context where genetic ties provide the cultural material on which familial relations are built and made meaningful (Schneider 1984), why was AID, but not egg donation, seen as threatening marriage and family life? Why were physicians so nonchalant about recruiting sperm donors but more concerned about egg donors? Some of the answers lie in the dominant framing of AID via the politics of family, in comparison to the framing of IVF via the politics of life: the historical and cultural context in which these technologies emerged led to distinctly different public and professional controversies about their implications.

But another part of the answers lies in the paradox that genes and gametes are both highly significant and utterly insignificant in relation to gender and parentage. Their (in)significance depends on whether we look at the giver or receiver of gametes, and whether we look at sperm or egg donation. In medical constructions of AID, sperm donors easily parted with their own sperm and theoretically had little interest in any resulting children, although there were a few exceptions to this view. Yet infertile husbands were viewed as less easily accepting donor sperm and AID-created paternity. Practitioners wondered if husbands would reject a donor-conceived child as illegitimate or view the act of artificial insemination as the wife's adultery because she was technically bearing the child of another man. In artificial insemination, the impregnating, paternal role belonged to the sperm donor—or the (typically male) physician performing the procedure. Sperm was highly important, but it was also unimportant to men depending on their relationship to the situation. Legitimacy was also both attached and unattached to sperm: in the face of doubt about whose sperm caused the pregnancy, marriage has historically provided an accepted answer via the marital presumption of paternity. In the face of certainty that the sperm was from a donor, physicians carefully constructed a façade of biology paternity using secrecy and "white lies" on the birth certificate. This façade helped protect men from multiple possible threats to their masculinity: their status as a cuckold or the somewhat lesser stigma of adoptive fatherhood, both of which publicly declared that they had not impregnated their own wife.

In egg donation, though, something else was happening. "Desperate" infertile women readily accepted donor eggs to gestate and nurture, seemingly without threat to their femininity or maternity. In contrast to sperm donors, egg donors were constructed (with some exceptions) as more emotionally attached to their eggs as symbolic reproductive opportunities. Practitioners wondered if egg donors were atoning for past abortions, making up for a childless future, or thinking about the egg as a child-to-be. For the egg recipient, the donated egg was a missing reproductive piece she needed in pursuing biological motherhood. For the egg donor, it was a possible child she might have had. The femininity threat was understood as substantially less severe for infertile women using egg donation, compared to the masculinity threat for men using AID. The pregnancy of an infertile woman was not a façade. Furthermore, the true biological source of the egg mattered less to the social order. Women did not bestow legitimacy on their children (only fathers could do that), so (il)legitimacy was irrelevant to egg donation, even as it was central to early discussions of AID.

Another element I propose here is that egg donation was also viewed as less threatening to the repronormative family because it did not have the sexual connotation that sperm donation did. In egg donation, the transfer of gametes occurs between two women: the donor and the recipient. Egg donation between IVF patients and sisters is asexual, altruistic,[13] and medicalized through the surgical procedures used to obtain eggs and transfer embryos between bodies. Even when anonymous or stranger egg donors were used, the notion that the sharing of an egg between two women might be sexualized or erotic did not enter the imagination of physicians.[14] This clinical, asexual tenor is apparent in a pair of illustrations for donation methods in an article by Dr. Zev Rosenwaks, director of the Jones Institute for Reproductive Medicine (1987). In both illustrations, the egg recipient is fully embodied, wearing surgical drapes and a cap and lying face down, with her hips elevated for the embryo transfer. Drawings of her internal reproductive organs are imposed over her pelvis. The egg donor is represented by her reproductive organs in one illustration and by an oocyte in the other. The recipient's husband is represented in both by his sperm alone, with the first illustration showing the sperm in the donor's reproductive tract and the second showing the sperm with a "+" sign next to the image of the oocyte. Any potential sexual relationship between donor and husband is downplayed by their disembodied representations. In the illustration with the "+" sign, they are literally reduced to parts of a reproductive equation. The illustrations' accompanying elements—a petri dish, a catheter, surgical drapes, and dividing cells—encourage a medicalized, asexual interpretation of the donation process.

In AID, in direct contrast to egg donation, using an extramarital donor is potentially sexual. The heterosexual pair of the male donor and female recipient makes an imagined sexual relationship possible. Inserting donor sperm directly into the recipient woman's body through AI implies the conjugal, procreative act. This is seen overtly in Guttmacher's (1943, 585) discussion of AI: "I place the patient in the lithotomy position [lying on one's back with legs flexed at the hips] and elevate the hips. . . . [T]he semen [is] spurted into the canal in four or five thrusts of the plunger of the syringe, simulating the mechanism in normal ejaculation." Thus, beyond gender, these different interpretations of egg and sperm donation are also shaped by heterosexuality. The feminist scholar Adrienne Rich used the term "compulsory heterosexuality" to describe sexuality as a political institution that perpetuates the social invisibility of lesbian existence and creates a series of constraints and sanctions that "insured the coupling of women with men" (1980, 636). If women are understood only as heterosexual, the transfer of eggs between two women could not have the same sexually and socially disruptive power that donor sperm would have for heterosexual marriage. This interpretation is further underscored by the taboo against using male relatives for AID, compared to the acceptability of asking sisters to donate their eggs. This also brings us full circle, back to how we think culturally about maternity as asexual and nurturing and about paternity as sexual and procreative. Men impregnate; women have babies. Men are fathers by their seed; women are mothers by their womb.

However, the story does not end here. In the next chapter, I wade into the cultural hierarchies in place for maternity and collaborative reproduction, looking at maternal claims making in patient literature. If egg donation is the next best thing to natural reproduction, where does that leave embryo donation and gestational surrogacy? Does gestation always matter more than genetics for deciding who is the most authentic mother of a child? The plotline of maternity gets more complicated.

4

Contingent Maternities?

Maternal Claims Making in Collaborative Reproduction

In her poignant study of the personal experience of infertility, the nursing scholar Margarete Sandelowski described the phenomenon of "childwaiting" for infertile couples who turned to adoption to build their families. Noting an "essential difference between childbearing and childwaiting," her female interviewees described being "reduced" to feeling like expectant fathers because they were physically disconnected from their child-to-be (1993, 181). Sandelowski observed that this was "distinctively a woman's loss" (183), compared to the norms of embodied, expectant motherhood. Adoption typically severs biology fully from parenthood. But what happens when biology is only partly severed? Are egg and embryo donation socially and culturally understood as closer to "natural" reproduction because they both retain the embodied, gestational experience? Is gestational surrogacy more akin to "childwaiting" because the intended rearing mother is not pregnant? Under the dominant norms of biological, expectant motherhood, (how) are women who use collaborative reproduction legally, medically, and socially recognized as authentic mothers of their child-to-be? In this chapter, I examine contemporary forms of maternal claims making in egg and embryo donation and in gestational surrogacy.

If early professional thinking on egg donation saw it as innocuous for the egg recipient's legal and socially recognized maternity, how does the conversation change when we consider other forms of collaborative reproduction that fragment biological maternity in different ways?

As my point of entry, I analyze infertility patient literature developed for women and couples contemplating collaborative reproduction. I draw on content created by the ASRM, RESOLVE, Organon USA (Organon), and Freedom Fertility Pharmacy (Freedom Fertility). ASRM and RESOLVE are both highly recognized agenda-setting organizations (K. Andrews and Edwards 2004) in the social world of reproductive medicine. They employ public educational campaigns to promote awareness about infertility and reproductive medicine, and they engage in lobbying efforts to shape public policy about reproductive rights, access to reproductive health care, and scientific research related to matters about reproduction. In chapter 1, I introduced the ASRM by its prior names: the American Fertility Society and, prior to that, the American Society for the Study of Sterility. Its final official name change in 1994 reflected the "broadened scope" of the organization, which was moving beyond fertility and sterility to "the study and investigation of reproductive medicine as a whole" (Duka and DeCherney 1994, 14). In the twenty-first century, the ASRM continues to be recognized as the major professional association for U.S. reproductive medicine. Its organizational vision is "to be the nationally and internationally recognized leader for multidisciplinary information, education, advocacy and standards in the field of reproductive medicine" (ASRM 2016).

RESOLVE offers a different perspective, as a patient-centered organization for men and women experiencing infertility. Established in 1974 by a nurse struggling with her own infertility, RESOLVE has grown into a national network of patients and providers that offers support, education, and advocacy related to infertility. Its official mission is "to provide timely, compassionate support and information to people who are experiencing infertility and to increase awareness of infertility issues through public education and advocacy" (RESOLVE 2016a). Though ASRM and RESOLVE were developed to serve professionals and patients, respectively, from its initiation, RESOLVE "had a close relationship with . . . physicians and the [American Fertility] Society" (Duka and DeCherney 1994, 248).

I also examine two patient booklets widely used in the fertility industry.[1] These booklets were written by practitioners but published and distributed by two major pharmaceutical companies that have developed fertility drugs: Organon Pharmaceuticals USA, Inc. which was founded in 1937 (Bloomberg 2022); and Freedom Fertility, a pharmacy company founded in 1973 that describes itself as "America's leading fertility pharmacy" (Freedom Fertility 2022). Both Organon and Freedom Fertility have interests in generating consumer demand for their fertility products, especially since the U.S. fertility industry is primarily concentrated in a private medical market (Conrad and Leiter 2004). They also strategically partner with practitioners in reproductive medicine to add legitimacy and medical authority to the patient booklets. Despite the rather distinct professional, advocacy, and commercial interests of the organizations producing the patient literature, the materials were quite similar in terms of their latent and manifest content.

Through the medium of patient literature, organizations such as ASRM, RESOLVE, Organon, and Freedom Fertility help women construct and justify maternal relationships to collaboratively conceived children. I show that the content of the patient literature overwhelmingly frames maternity as a tension between genetics and gestation but also sides with one or the other, depending on the intended audience and technique being discussed. Egg donation patients read that their wombs are the ultimate source of maternal connection to their child, while surrogacy patients are told that their genetic connection is the linchpin of their maternity. This is likely strategically intended to create more willing patient-consumers and assuage anxieties about using potentially deviant technologies for family building. Yet I also show that the emphasized tension between eggs and wombs overshadows and obscures the situational aspects of maternity through collaborative reproduction—what I call here 'contingent maternities.' Contingent maternities require that a constellation of factors be aligned for maternity to be fully recognized. I also specifically show that adding embryo donation to the analysis helps us move beyond the simple dichotomy of eggs versus wombs and illuminates the broader situation: embryo donation exposes the crucial fact that (partnered heterosexual) women's maternal claims are shored up by their partner's paternity claims. Thus, biologically fragmented maternity is not presented as a truly autonomous form of maternity. Instead, the various possible maternities resulting from collaborative reproduction are highly contingent and, therefore, potentially discreditable (Goffman 1963).

Making Kin, Making Mothers

In thinking about multiple possible maternities and maternal claims making, I draw on the rich body of prior literature that uses the ideas of 'doing kinship' and 'doing family,' some of which has made its way into scholarly thinking about the new reproductive technologies (e.g., Thompson 2005; Teman 2010). According to this social constructionist perspective, family and kinship are both ideas and relationships that are continuously constituted and made meaningful in everyday actions, as opposed to a natural, predetermined order assumed to emerge from biology (Gubrium and Holstein 1993; Holstein and Gubrium 1999; Nelson 2006; Smith 1993). Maternal claims making is one part of the work of doing kinship but is often invisible, arising in situations where maternity is uncertain or disputed. I define maternal claims making here as the activity of articulating and justifying a moral, legal, or social claim to a particular child. From the viewpoint of the repronormative family, maternal claims making assumes that there is one ultimate mother who has the strongest, most authentic claim to a child. This assumption is openly refuted in some family forms, such as co-maternity among lesbian couples who both intentionally contribute biologically to a child to assert dual maternity, one providing the eggs and the other gestating. More generally, claims making is a persuasive activity (Best 1987). At its core, maternal claims making recognizes that maternity, like other familial relationships, is not necessarily an objective and uncontested fact but must be expressed to be recognized (Holstein and Gubrium 1999).

Prior research on surrogacy has focused on maternity and maternal claiming. Elly Teman (2010, 110) showed how Israeli surrogates and intended mothers both downplayed the surrogate and affirmed the intended mother through "maternal claiming," which referred to "techniques aimed at claiming entitlement to the social label of mother of the expected baby." Heather Jacobson (2016, 90) found that many U.S. surrogates were reluctant to work with intended mothers who were not using their own eggs because their insecurities about maternity created "an extra layer of [emotional] labor." Addressing U.S. egg donation and surrogacy, Charis Thompson (2005, 148) identified "relational" versus "custodial" stages of reproduction, noting that the former "can support claims of parenthood," while the latter "involve[s] caring for the gametes or embryos . . . [but] cannot sustain parental claims." Thompson also noted resources used to strategically naturalize the intended mother's maternity: biology, sociocultural taboos (e.g., the incest taboo, which prevents a sister donor or surrogate from having her male sibling's child), and "procreative intent" (148) (i.e., who pays for treatment, who the gametes and embryos originate from or technically belong to, whose partner provides the sperm, and who has future child-rearing responsibility). Amrita Pande's (2009) work showed how Indian gestational surrogates claimed kinship to a surrogate-born child through shared bodily substances of blood (nourishment through gestation), sweat (from the labor of gestation), and breast milk (if a surrogate did the breast-feeding). Yet Pande distinctly identified these as kinship and not maternal claims, concluding that "everyday forms of kinship . . . [likely] pose very little threat to the fundamental (genetic) basis of establishing kin ties" (393). Thus, such kinship claims did not disturb the intended mother's maternity claim.

This prior work provides important insights into the individual and interpersonal processes of identity work in kinship and maternal claims making, emphasizing the voices of patients or intended parents, donors, and surrogates. My goal here is to shift the focus from these interactions and put the organizational discourse at the forefront. The social world of reproductive medicine does not simply provide tools and components to assist reproduction. It actively shapes, channels, and produces families, in concert with cultural ideas about what families should look like. This represents one example of what the sociologists Jaber Gubrium and James Holstein (1993) described as the "organizational embeddedness" of families and family life. Contemporary family life and familial relationships are made meaningful in and through organizations that offer various human services. These organizations reflect, create, and reconstitute the social order.

Organizations are also affected by the broader norms of the social and cultural environment in which they exist. For example, in response to changing norms about families as well as mounting evidence from social science, the ASRM Ethics Committee (2006a) stated that gay, lesbian, and unmarried people should not be barred from receiving fertility services. The committee urged practitioners to accept patients "without regard to marital status or sexual orientation" (1333). This was a major shift from the ethical stance of this committee's predecessor, the AFS Committee on Ethics (1986, 1990, and 1994), that married heterosexual couples provided the best foundation for family building. At the same time, reproductive medicine has a long history of aiming to (re)-create the repronormative family (Agigian 2004; Haimes 1993a), and change toward accepting more diverse patients and family forms is uneven (Johnson 2012). Actors and organizations in reproductive medicine therefore straddle different ideologies of the family. They sell innovative products and services as well as new forms of fragmented maternity as therapies for infertility, but they are also culturally inculcated in the repronormative family ideal.

Framing Patient Expectations

ASRM, RESOLVE, Organon, and Freedom Fertility have distinct organizational goals, which influence their patient literature.

As a professional medical organization, ASRM seeks to educate patients about medical procedures, including the risks and benefits of different assisted reproductive methods. Its patient literature is overtly scientific in tone and full of medical jargon. RESOLVE is a patient-centered organization that focuses more explicitly on social and emotional support. Its literature contains many personal anecdotes and focuses more on social and psychological issues related to the infertility experience and its treatment. As for-profit corporations, both Organon and Freedom Fertility are interested in generating consumer demand for their fertility products. The patient literature they produce and sponsor is intended to increase their legitimacy and elevate their status with patients, and it is created in collaboration with practitioners in reproductive medicine. But who they collaborate with affects the content of the literature. For instance, the Organon booklet is written by two reproductive endocrinologists and primarily addresses the medical procedure of egg donation, with its risks and benefits (Doody and Sauer 2000). On the front cover is a picture of a woman in a contemplative pose, with an image of an oocyte directly below, as viewed under a microscope. The only other images in the booklet are sample screening forms and a timeline displaying the process of synchronizing donors and recipients. The booklet uses a medical and scientific tone throughout. In contrast, the Freedom Fertility booklet was developed by a reporter who covered health and medicine topics in the New England region, a clinical psychologist affiliated with a fertility clinic, and a clinical nursing director for multiple donor egg programs (Birrittieri, Fusillo, and Witkin n.d.). The content focuses primarily on social and emotional aspects of egg donation. The cover shows a white heterosexual couple, laughing and hugging. Images of heterosexual couples (both white and Asian) appear throughout the pamphlet, with the couples in close and embracing postures that signify emotional connection and intimate relations. Both the Organon and Freedom Fertility booklets are general resources that many fertility clinics include in patient packets for oocyte recipients.

All four organizations have an interest in encouraging the use of collaborative reproduction. While they do so in different ways (e.g., appealing to affect versus science or technology), they collectively work to normalize biologically fragmented maternity. One major 'elephant in the room' that they have to recognize and reckon with is the dominant maternal ideal of integrated bio-social-legal maternity. Indeed, throughout the patient literature, regardless of source, both genetic and gestational ties to a child is considered the most authentic form of maternity. This reflects and reinforces a cultural hierarchy of motherhood in which "biological motherhood is more highly valued than social motherhood . . . enable[ing] a woman to fulfill herself in terms of expected biological and social roles" (Letherby 1999, 367). While using collaborative reproduction allows for an approximation of authentic maternity, it also falls short. In this vein, these various reproductive organizations were not trying to replace the old hierarchy of maternity with a new order. Rather, they were trying to weave collaborative reproduction into the old hierarchy, describing it as at least partially compatible with, and made intelligible through, existing ideas about maternity.

Discussing the emotional aspects of collaborative reproduction, that author of one RESOLVE article observed that the techniques can offer "the possibility of being pregnant" as well as "having a child who has a genetic connection to one of its parents" (Dolinsky 2009). This article initially framed collaborative reproduction in a positive light. However, one of the first emotional issues covered in the article was grieving "the loss of the child and family you imagined having the traditional way." Notably, this grief was not about the actual loss of a child or family but about accepting the fact that collaborative reproduction was low in the "reproductive hierarchy" (Bell 2019, 483).

Among collaborative forms of reproduction, there is also a second hierarchy to confront: a hierarchy of which techniques are considered more acceptable to use among the different options (Letherby 1999). Both egg donation and gestational surrogacy "threaten 'ideal' motherhood" (368). However, egg donation is considered closer to natural pregnancy—an idea that also surfaced in the way practitioners initially thought about egg donation (as discussed in chapter 3). This second hierarchy also clearly comes through in the patient literature. For example, the Organon booklet described egg donation pregnancy as "progress[ing] normally" after the first trimester, when it no longer needed to be sustained by externally administered hormones: "following delivery, mothers often breastfeed, no different than with spontaneous conception" (Doody and Sauer 2000, 3). This language emphasizes the normalness and naturalness of a pregnancy involving egg donation. Although collaborative and traditional reproduction diverge in initial conception and early pregnancy, they are the same during pregnancy, labor and delivery, and the postpartum period. Taking another tack to elevate egg donation in this hierarchy of maternity options, the Freedom Fertility booklet distanced egg donation from both adoption and surrogacy, noting that "egg donation is not a form of adoption" but rather a "natural experience" that allows women to have their own "biological child" (Birrittieri et al. n.d., 4).

While egg donation is firmly elevated to the top of the hierarchy of collaborative reproduction, gestational surrogacy was demoted below egg donation, described as a less desirable option than carrying the baby oneself. The author of a RESOLVE article on "Myths about Surrogates/Gestational Carriers" noted: "A woman often chooses surrogacy after numerous attempts and methods to conceive and a carry a baby herself" (Williams 2011). Another RESOLVE article, titled "Surrogacy," similarly affirmed that surrogacy was "seldom the first choice on the journey to build a family" (RESOLVE 2016e). In the introduction to the ASRM patient guide on third-party reproduction, the authors explicitly noted that surrogacy was more "controversial" than egg donation and was "subject to both legal and psychosocial scrutiny," thereby presenting it as a less appealing option (ASRM 2012, 3). However, the authors also noted that gestational surrogacy was "legally . . . a lower-risk procedure" than traditional surrogacy and therefore was more commonly used in the United States. The message was quite clear: having some biological connection to one's child was legally, psychologically, and socially better than having none.

Embryo donation sits somewhere in limbo in the hierarchy of collaborative reproduction options. It is likened to gamete donation in some instances and to traditional adoption in others, because both the egg and sperm are typically donated by a second heterosexual couple who have excess embryos after undergoing their own fertility treatments. However, much of the patient literature made it clear that in many cases embryo donation was still "preferable to [traditional] adoption" (RESOLVE 2016b). While couples receiving donated embryos may still have to come to terms with "disappointment" and "emotional distress" over not having their "own genetic child," the procedure still allows them to experience pregnancy and childbirth in their journey to parenthood.[2]

In a personal narrative on the RESOLVE website, "Maggie" and her husband, "Frank," tried to have a baby "without success for several years" (RESOLVE 2016c). They first "sought the advice of a local fertility specialist." After learning that all of their IVF-created embryos had "genetic problems," they looked into both egg donation and traditional adoption. Later, they learned about embryo donation, through which they ended up having two children. Although the reader is not told why they decided against egg donation, embryo donation clearly ranked above adoption for them as a family-building option. Through "Mary's Story," also on the RESOLVE website, we learn about a couple who had excess IVF-created embryos after going through their own infertility struggles (RESOLVE 2016d). They opted to donate these to another infertile couple. The receiving couple did not have a successful pregnancy with the donated embryos. However, going through the embryo donation process helped "open" them to adoption, and they later adopted two children. Adoption was clearly their last resort, and receiving donated embryos was a step on the path to accepting it, helping loosen their commitment to achieving biological parenthood.

Multiple hierarchies—those of motherhood, reproduction, and acceptable reproductive techniques (Bell 2019; Letherby 1999; Wegar 1997)—show which techniques are framed as socially and culturally acceptable, and in which order they should be tried, when attempts to have fully biological children are unsuccessful. Given such hierarchies and the tenuousness of partial biology, how are women using each specific collaborative technique recognized as authentic mothers of their child-to-be?

Egg Donation and Gestational or Embodied Maternal Claims

Maternal claims through egg donation are rooted in the experience of pregnancy and childbirth. This most closely mimics the legal tradition of recognizing the birth mother as the 'true' mother of a child (Kindregan 2009; Stumpf 1986). In chapter 3, I showed how early physicians and nonmedical critics and experts viewed egg donation as more natural than surrogacy or adoption, precisely because egg donation did not disturb the biological presumption of maternity. However, the patient literature on egg donation used a different tactic, first explicitly separating the genetic and gestational components of maternity and then elevating gestation over genetics as representing a more authentic maternal claim to a child. Notably, several authors used the term "biology," as opposed to "gestational" or "pregnancy," to refer to gestational maternity. The strategic lack of specificity of the term "biology" allows it to be more flexible and overarching.

For example, the ASRM patient guide on third-party reproduction noted that an egg recipient would have "a biological but not genetic relationship to the child" (ASRM 2012, 4). Intriguingly, this was followed by the claim that "her partner (if he provided the sperm) will be both biologically and genetically related." As men have no other biological connection to a child beyond their genetic contribution, the use of "biological" to describe both maternal and paternal connections in egg donation pregnancies implies that biology is more important and more encompassing than mere genetics.

In a RESOLVE article addressing "Donors' Attitudes about Egg Donation," Hilary Marshak, a social worker specializing in infertility counseling described her years of experience addressing intended parents' anxiety that the child will not feel that the "[egg recipient] birthmother is his or her 'real' mother" (Marshak 2009)—referring to culturally salient ideas about adoptive versus birth parents (Wegar 1998), but with a twist that instead pitted birth mother against genetic mother. Marshak noted, however, that "once [prenatal] bonding has occurred, it becomes a non-issue," stressing the embodied physical, psychological, and social experience of pregnancy as the source of maternity making for women using egg donation. Notably, the pamphlet only addressed the intended mother's anxiety about how the donor-conceived child would feel, not the actual feelings of the imagined child. But the author also suggested that pregnancy would nullify the latter problem as well, making any forthcoming family discussions about maternity a "non-issue."

The biological versus genetic distinction also appears in the introduction to the Freedom Fertility booklet. One of the authors, a clinical psychologist working in a fertility clinic, observed that "day after day" she "help[s] couples understand the difference between 'genetic' and 'biological' contribution" (Birrittieri et al n.d., 3). She helped couples understand "that a donor egg simply delivers some genetic material to help them conceive a child of their own." The message here is that genetics are necessary but insufficient to create a child. Importantly, the lack of a genetic connection does not interfere with the intended mother's claiming the child as her "own." The authors went on to assert that the maternal connection was created through the embodied, life-generating experience of pregnancy (Birrittieri et al. n.d.):

The implanted embryo builds its body from its mother's body. (5)

Many believe the uterus is simply an incubator. . . . The most important aspect of all pregnancies—including egg donation pregnancies—is that as the fetus grows, every cell in the developing body is built from the pregnant mother's body. (9)

You, as their mother, are their source of life. (23)

In these descriptions, the maternal body is the all-encompassing provider of the raw materials for the child-to-be. The initial genetic input is minuscule compared to the gestational labor of building and nurturing the fetal body.

While the egg donation patient literature elevated the embodied, gestational experience as the ultimate maternal connection, it also had to downplay the lack of genetic connection to assert women's sole maternal claim to a child. The authors of the Organon booklet referred in passing to an egg donor as a "genetic mother," putting quotation marks around the term (Doody and Sauer 2000, 8). This seems to acknowledge that the donor's maternal status was contested but also to suggest that there was no other language readily available to describe her reproductive contribution. In the RESOLVE article on egg donor attitudes, noted above, social worker Marshak (2009) observed that many intended parents would be comforted by knowing that in her years of counseling potential egg donors, she had found that many viewed their egg donations as analogous to "donating an organ" and their eggs as being "just [human] tissue," and that they otherwise had no "attachment to [their] eggs." This statement implied that genetics had little significance to the donor and therefore did not stand in the way of the gestational mother's maternal claim. Notably, this position was also a decided shift from earlier professional views on egg donors as being emotionally attached to their eggs (as discussed in chapter 3). In an interesting discursive move, the authors of the Freedom Fertility booklet effectively removed genetic maternity from the reproductive equation, stating that "with egg donation, the child has always had only two parents, the biological mother, and the genetic father" (Birrittieri et al. n.d., 19). Filling both roles of the two-parent, repronormative family closed off the possibility of any maternal claims making by the egg donor.

Despite generally downplaying the importance of genetics for maternal claims making, much of the patient literature on egg donation emphasized that women would likely need to grieve about or be counseled on the loss of a genetic connection to their child: "You've tried so hard. You're overwhelmed and emotionally bankrupt. . . . Take time for yourself when you have exhausted the traditional means of conceiving. . . . If your doctor reports that you need an egg donor, you may grieve about losing the genetic link to your child. Take time to process this loss" (Dreyfus n.d.). This notion of grief over losing a chance at fully integrated, biological maternity also reasserted its cultural significance: stoking an ember of maternity uncertainty about gestational-only maternal claims.

Gestational Surrogacy and Genetic Claims

If the primary authentic maternal claim in egg donation is the embodied, gestational experience, what does this leave in cases of gestational surrogacy, where the intended mother uses her egg but does not carry the pregnancy? How can gestational surrogacy be reconciled with gestational maternity as the "source of life" for the growing fetus? In direct contradiction to the framing of egg donation, maternal claims making in gestational surrogacy was rooted in the genetic tie to the intended mother's egg. However, maternity via gestational surrogacy was also framed as more tenuous than maternity via egg donation. In light of this, the patient literature offered additional strategies for intended mothers to bolster their maternal claims and also used language that symbolically minimized the competing maternal claims of the surrogate.

While the patient literature recognized that women using egg donation might need to be reconciled to the loss of their own genetic contribution to their child, one positive aspect of gestational surrogacy was that it offered a way to maintain the genetic family. In a RESOLVE (2016e) article titled "Surrogacy," we read the story of "Sharon" and "Dan"—a couple that had endured "three miscarriages and years of infertility." After Sharon found out she could not "carry a baby," the couple explored "adoption and resolving [to live] without children," but Sharon was reluctant to "give up her dream of having children." Through looking into the different family-building options, Dan also came to realize his "own deep desire" to have "a child who will carry on the traits of my family." Dan wanted a child "who might be blessed with my mom's musical talents or have my dad's sparkly eyes." Gestational surrogacy gave them the opportunity to come as close as possible to "having our child in the 'usual' way"—referring to the normative hierarchy of reproduction. Later, under the heading "Emotional Considerations," the article addressed the importance of couples' receiving adequate counseling before surrogacy, especially to explore how they felt about "someone else carrying your child." The idea of someone else carrying their child reinforced the unnaturalness of the gestational surrogacy arrangement, but this was countered by the possessive pronoun "your,"—emphasizing the intended parents' connection and claim to the child. Some readers might interpret this possessive language as constructing embryos as property of the genetic contributors, which is a contested position ethically and legally (L. Andrews 1986b; Berg 2005). I suggest instead that the possessive language indicates a moral claiming of the child-to-be, identifying its family group membership, identity, and belonging. Finally, the last counseling question for couples to consider was: "how will you explain the pregnancy and birth to others and eventually to your child?" (RESOLVE 2016e). This reinforced the deviation of gestational surrogacy from the traditional story of biosocial reproduction. 'Natural' reproduction, on the other hand, needs no such explanation.

Overall, the patient literature portrayed maternal claims in surrogacy as more tenuous than the gestational, embodied connection in egg donation. As a result, the claims in surrogacy required additional support to bolster them, such as reinforcing the proximity of the intended mother to the pregnancy and downplaying the role of the surrogate, strategies that both Thompson (2005) and Teman (2010) described in their research on surrogacy and collaborative reproduction. In an example of reinforcing the intended mother's proximity to the pregnancy, a RESOLVE article described surrogacy as "sharing a pregnancy with a carrier" and an option that allowed the intended mother to be "involve[d] with the pregnancy and prenatal care . . . and being present for the birth of your child" (RESOLVE 2016e). While the "involvement" with pregnancy and prenatal care allowed the intended mother to share in the experience, the notion of "sharing a pregnancy" discursively joined the reproductive experience of the intended mother and gestational surrogate, making it sound as if they were both simultaneously pregnant. The notion of proximity to the pregnancy also came through in Sharon and Dan's story cited above. Sharon described how she came to accept surrogacy: "I realized I could have a genetic child and be very close to the pregnancy even if I wasn't carrying the child myself" (RESOLVE 2016e). She went on to describe the experience of the first ultrasound and seeing "my child's heartbeat." By maintaining physical and social proximity to the pregnancy through attending prenatal appointments, Sharon could engage in some of the same rituals as other expectant mothers. This helps close the gap between the distant "childwaiting" of traditional adoption (Sandelowski 1993) and the rituals of expectant motherhood that center on encounters with the fetus, both inside and through the maternal body—such as hearing the fetal heartbeat, viewing the anatomy scan, learning the fetal sex, and feeling fetal movements.

The second key strategy used to bolster women's maternal claims involved minimizing the role of the surrogate. Teman (2010) and Zsuzsa Berend (2016) both observed how surrogates themselves used language that reduced them from women to machines or body parts, attempting to limit the possibility of their being defined as the mother. Much feminist scholarship on surrogacy has decried this construction of surrogacy as dehumanizing and objectifying—a core part of the rationale for viewing surrogacy as oppressive for women (Rothman 1989; Lublin 1998; Thompson 2002). The patient literature also relied on these minimizing and objectifying strategies to distance the surrogate role from the maternal role. For example, throughout the ASRM literature, the authors noticeably avoided the phrase "surrogate mother." Instead, they described the surrogate as a "gestational carrier," "gestational surrogate," or "carrier" (see for example, ASRM 2011 and 2012). The RESOLVE article on "Surrogacy" referred to gestational surrogacy as "gestational care" (RESOLVE 2016e), making the arrangement sound more like prenatal child care than pregnancy—which is indeed how some surrogates view their surro-pregnancy (Berend 2016). In RESOLVE's "Questions to Ask Series," the very person-hood of the surrogate disappeared, as the only terms used were "gestational surrogacy," "surrogacy IVF," and (most telling) "host uterus" (RESOLVE 2016f). The latter term discursively reduced the surrogate from a whole woman, who might have maternal desires for the fetus she was carrying, to a reproductive organ.[3] This directly contradicts the claim in the patient literature about egg donation that the gestational contribution was to be not simply an "incubator" but an all-encompassing life source for the child-to-be.

In seeming contradiction to the minimizing strategy, other patient literature emphasized the uniqueness of the surrogate and the need for her to "mesh" with the couple (Dreyfus n.d.). For instance, the author of "Choosing between Egg Donor and Surrogate" noted (Dreyfus n.d.): "finding the right surrogate mom" is "beyond important." She then tells the story of one married intended mother meeting her surrogate: "We instantly fell in love with her!" and "I felt like I was hugging my own sister" (quoted in Dreyfus n.d.).[4] Here, the surrogate's personhood was crucial to creating a successful arrangement. Yet her role was also strategically located as like that of a sister. Positioning her in this way helps sidestep any maternal claims she might have. At most she might claim to be like an aunt. Providing this alternate kinship role for the surrogate can strategically minimize her maternal claims, preventing her from competing with the intended mother.

Embryo Donation and the Transfer of Parentage

Although embryo donation should theoretically be analogous to egg donation because the intended mother can make maternal claims through the embodied experience of pregnancy and childbirth, such claims appeared even more tenuous than maternal claims in either egg donation or gestational surrogacy. This was grounded in two facts: neither intended parent of the presumedly heterosexual recipient couple had a genetic connection to the embryo and both members of another heterosexual couple retained genetic ties via a conjugal embryo.[5] Here even gestational, embodied motherhood was trumped by the existence of two other genetic parents in a socially recognized heterosexual relationship with one another. For instance, a RESOLVE brochure for embryo recipient couples suggested that embryo donation might be sought by a couple to "eliminate the imbalance when only one member of a couple loses the genetic connection to their children" (RESOLVE n.d.a, 2). Yet the significance of losing both genetic ties was reaffirmed later in the brochure, where counseling issues included discussing "feelings and fears about parenting a child *created by another couple*" (3, my emphasis). The ASRM patient fact sheet on embryo donation described having recipient couples counseled about "nonbiologic parentage" (ASRM 2012b)—implicitly overlooking the possibility that intended mothers might have biological ties through gestation.

The tenacity of the genetic connection in embryo donation was further emphasized through personal stories from RESOLVE. For "Mary" and her husband (unnamed)—a couple with excess embryos after infertility treatment—it was important to have a say in "selecting" the recipient couple (RESOLVE 2016d). Mary described how she and her husband talked to the recipient couple over the phone to get a "sense of who they were as people" and to be "comfortable with their decision." Mary and her husband were not simply providing cells for a medical procedure. Rather, they were entrusting the recipient couple with their embryos: embryos that might have become their own children.

The story of "Maggie" and "Frank" (RESOLVE 2016c) provides the perspective of a couple that received embryos from three different donating couples. The first arrangement was with a known donor couple, but the pregnancy was unsuccessful. The latter two donations were anonymous arrangements: Maggie and Frank learned about the donating couples through reading profiles of potential donors. Then they ended up having two children from these anonymous donations. Maggie and Frank also decided that if they had any excess embryos after treatment they would return them to the "donor pool" to help another "potential family" (RESOLVE 2016c). This suggested that they viewed the embryos as fungible biological material—a resource needed to create children, as opposed to children-to-be of the specific donating couples. However, this perspective was likely bolstered by the fact that they did not speak with or meet the donating couples. Maggie's and Frank's parentage claims to their embryo-donor-conceived children were supported by the anonymity of the arrangements. Furthermore, since they were receiving the embryos, framing the embryos as a biological resource allowed them to build up their own familial and parentage claims, while downplaying the significance of the conjugal embryos they received.

Given that the genetic ties of the donating couple appear to have greater weight in embryo donation than in egg donation, and that gestation does not have the same elevated status, women's maternal claims in this situation were framed primarily through the contractual transfer of parentage to the recipient couple and the "commitment the [intended] parents have made to gestate the embryo" (ASRM 2012a, 13). Both the ASRM and RESOLVE literature emphasized the need to have proper agreements in place to recognize parentage transfers through embryo donation. This framed parentage as a matter of rights and responsibilities as opposed to something rooted in a biological connection to the child:

All your rights to the embryos and any offspring resulting from embryo donation will be relinquished. (RESOLVE n.d.b, 2)

[You will a]ssume full responsibility for all donated embryos as well as any resulting children. (RESOLVE n.d.a, 3)

Where there is little legal precedent regarding the use of donor embryos [the ASRM] recommends that the recipient accept full responsibility for the transferred embryo(s) and resulting children. (ASRM 2012b)

This emphasis on the contractual transfer of parentage indicates that even though women still had access to gestational or embodied maternal claims through embryo donation, the lack of a genetic tie on the part of both partners in the recipient couple destabilized gestation as a solid path to maternal claims making. Embodied maternity here still needed to be reinforced through both agreements to transfer parental rights between donating and receiving couples and the recognition of procreative intent through the recipient couples' "commitment" to gestating the embryo. Maternity through embryo donation was treated as more akin to adoption than to another form of biological (fragmented) maternity.

A Newly Contingent Maternity?

Gestational surrogacy, egg donation, and embryo donation have been in use for several decades, but the fragmented maternities that these techniques produce continue to challenge common legal and cultural assumptions about what makes someone a mother. Previous research has shown how both recipients or intended mothers and donors or surrogates employ various strategies to reconfigure the infertility patient as the 'true' mother and downplay parental claims of donors or surrogates (Thompson 2005; Teman 2010; Jacobson 2016). In this chapter, I focused on patient literature about collaborative reproduction. I examined how four different organizations in the social world of reproductive medicine offered constructions of maternity when biological ties were fragmented through using egg donation, gestational surrogacy, or embryo donation. Prior work on doing kinship and maternal claiming primarily focused on individual and interpersonal identity work. Therefore, one aim of my analysis was to examine the role of organizations in this identity work, contributing to the literature on how family roles and relationships are conceived in and through organizations that offer human and family services (Gubrium and Holstein 1993). Notably, the organizations examined here are agenda setters (K. Andrews and Edwards 2004) in U.S. reproductive medicine. While they do not use all of the ways in which fragmented maternity is understood, they are major figures in creating and disseminating patient literature and therefore dominate the discursive constructions of maternity via collaborative reproduction. They also lobby state and federal governments to influence law and policy decisions about reproductive medicine and technology. Their discursive constructions of family and maternity do not just circulate in the symbolic realm but can also have material impacts on families' lives.

The patient literatures on gestational surrogacy and egg donation stand in direct contradiction to one another regarding which maternal tie is given primacy: genetics versus gestation. Both literatures assert that the emphasized tie offers an accepted path to motherhood, with caveats. Maternal claims in egg donation are achieved by elevating the role of gestational or embodied motherhood through the intended mother's experience of pregnancy, childbirth, and breast-feeding, as well as downplaying the role and significance of genetics. In gestational surrogacy, genetic ties are emphasized as the primary pathway. However, intended mothers need to support their maternal claims by engaging in additional activities that could fulfill the social rituals of expectant motherhood and minimizing the role of the surrogate's body. The latter strategy is clearly seen through the description of surrogacy as a "host uterus"—which effectively removes the personhood of the surrogate and thereby any of her competing claims to maternity. Although embryo donation seems to be analogous to egg donation, with intended mothers able to make maternal claims through the biological, embodied connection of pregnancy, this is not the tactic used. Embryo donation is framed as a significantly riskier procedure, and in one case the potential child is described as a "child created by another couple," making it discursively closer to adoption than to other forms of biological parenthood. Two points become apparent in the literature on embryo donation: neither genetics nor gestation are presented as uniquely sufficient for establishing maternity, and not only women's biological ties but also the genetic ties of their male partners are important in establishing maternity.

This allows us to see how women's claims to maternity in both egg donation and surrogacy are further stabilized by them being in a heterosexual relationship with the genetic father. For example, if we revisit some of the patient literature quoted above on egg donation, we learn that the child conceived through egg donation has only ever had "two parents, the biological mother, and the genetic father." This fact of genetic fatherhood, although seemingly secondary to the biological mother in this case, serves to reinforce her maternal claims by filling both roles of the presumed two-parent, heterosexual family. Similarly, if we revisit Sharon and Dan's story, we see that they refer to surrogacy as providing a close approximation of "having our child in the 'usual' way." Additionally, that article described the process of surrogacy as "someone else carrying your child." Implied by this is that the wife's claim to maternity is not just through using her egg and having that genetic connection. Rather, it is reinforced by her relationship to the genetic father of the child. The child is considered 'theirs' because its genetic origin is cemented in the context of the nuclear, heterosexual family. The conjugal embryo refers back to and reinforces the repronormative family.

The need to reinforce biologically fragmented maternal claims points to underlying norms that likely permeate ASRM, RESOLVE, Organon, and Freedom Fertility. Family building through assisted and collaborative reproduction does not occur in a cultural vacuum, but in relation to broader discourses about families. In particular, the repronormative family acts as a cultural resource, framing norms and assumptions in the patient literature to organize fragmented maternal claims and make them intelligible. Without the various pieces—asserting a primary maternal claim, downplaying competing claims, and establishing a maternal-paternal conjugal relationship—women's maternity status is potentially destabilized and thus socially, legally, or psychologically discreditable (Goffman 1963). In his classic work on stigma, Erving Goffman distinguishes between the discredited individual, whose "differentness" is already known or easily perceivable, and the potentially discreditable person, whose "differentness is not immediately apparent, and is not known beforehand" (1963, 42). The latter individual is burdened with the task of choosing whether "to display or not to display; to tell or not to tell; to let on or not to let on; to lie or not to lie; and in each case, to whom, how, when, and where." The status of biological maternity is not easily perceivable, except in cases of a significant discrepancy in the outward appearances of mother and child. At the same time, the intended mother's status is potentially socially and legally tenuous, if the donor or surrogate were to assert maternal claims and state laws lacked clarity or did not overtly favor the intended mother. Additionally, as several surrogates mentioned in Jacobson's study (2016), intended mothers may feel insecure in their maternal claims, not having personally reconciled the disparity between the fully integrated, biological maternity that is culturally expected and the biologically fragmented maternity available to them.

Thus, I suggest that the newer forms of maternity available via collaborative reproduction are framed as highly situational and relationally constructed as opposed to being based strictly in either genetic or gestational claims. Rather than maternity based on its own autonomous foundation, these are contingent maternities—forms of maternity established through carefully constructed arrangements that can be challenged. Indeed, although egg or embryo recipients and intended social mothers of surrogacy-born children can articulate distinct maternal claims to their children, they are at risk of not being assigned maternity. As Teman (2010, 5) observed about gestational surrogacy. "an intended mother faces the reality that another woman is carrying her baby [and] potentially has a privileged claim to social recognition as the baby's mother."

In chapters 3 and 4, I have explored perspectives on collaborative reproduction and maternity within the social world of reproductive medicine. Medicine creates the scientific and technological possibilities for new maternities, but law regulates which families become formally recognized as authentic social units, endowed with rights and responsibilities to their members. In the next two chapters, I wade into the social world of law as it intersects with collaborative reproduction and parentage. Sorting out maternity in contested situations further shows how the work of maternal claims making has material implications for families. In particular, some definitions and pathways to maternity are considered more authentic in light of the notion of the repronormative family. The steps taken to regulate collaborative reproduction shows how states grapple with redefining or reinforcing the natural family, with definitions of maternity and the maternal-child bond often at the center of emerging controversies.

5

Designating Maternity

Contested Motherhood and the Courts

In February 2009, Carolyn and Sean Savage attended an IVF appointment to have some of their frozen embryos implanted in the hope of having a younger sibling for their twins. Carolyn conceived a singleton pregnancy. Just over a week later, the Savages received a call from the clinic, informing them of a "terrible error" (Seewer 2009). There had been a mix-up, and the clinician had implanted the wrong embryo in Carolyn's uterus. A day later, Shannon and Paul Morell received a similar phone call. It was their embryo that the clinic had accidentally transferred to Carolyn Savage. Both couples were upset by the news and unsure how to proceed. As devout Catholics, the Savages did not want to seek an abortion, despite their doctor's advice. Carolyn opted to carry the pregnancy to term, and she and Sean decided that "the right thing—the only thing—to do was to give the baby to the biological parents" (Seewer 2009). Carolyn gave birth in late September, with the Morells "waiting down the hall" for their genetic son. Sean Savage described "the very short walk" down the hall to the Morells as "exceptionally emotional . . . but at the same time there was a sense of pride . . . that what we were doing was right" (quoted in Seewer 2009). Both couples suffered loss from the mix-up. The Savages lost the opportunity for Carolyn to have a future pregnancy because of her health. They would need to use a surrogate for any future genetic children. Carolyn also suffered from post-traumatic stress after the birth, despite feeling that it was the right thing to do to give the baby to the Morells (Fox 2019). The Morells lost out on the birth experience, the social bonding and rituals of pregnancy, and embodied expectant parenthood. They also no longer felt absolutely secure in their rights to the custody and legal parentage of their genetic child. The clinic error biologically and emotionally entangled the lives of people who had been strangers. The Savage-Morell story concludes with the different parties disambiguating parentage among themselves, remaking order from the initial confusion. Readers can understand the immense suffering everyone involved experienced because of the mistake. Some likely feel a sense of relief to learn that the child successfully delivered back to the Morells as the original, intended parents, while others might feel that this was an injustice to the Savages.

IVF has created numerous possibilities for solving or circumventing problems of infertility. But as the above story shows, it also has elements of risk and uncertainty. In this chapter, I focus on how partially disembodied reproductive techniques produce this uncertainty, looking at situations of contested maternity after an IVF mix-up. While the Savage-Morell case was resolved amicably without legal intervention, other situations have ended with terminated pregnancies or relied on the courts to adjudicate parentage claims (Bender 2006; Fox 2019). I focus here on two embryo mix-up cases in the United States that went to court. Both cases involved the mistaken transfer of embryos into the wrong patient's uterus at IVF clinics. The underlying issues in these cases, similar to the Savage-Morell story, is the need to place the embryo or resulting child with its natural parents, primarily by identifying maternity. Yet there are no definitive guidelines that can be used to quickly and easily sort out unintentionally fragmented maternity.

In the absence of legal clarity, state courts are tasked with designating maternity. Maternity designation occurs all the time, but it often goes unnoticed in the smooth transition from biological to legal parentage. A woman gives birth, and that act is unquestioned evidence of her maternity. She fills out paperwork for the child's birth certificate and social security card, with help from the hospital. Her maternity—never in question in the first place—becomes formally recognized by law. However, the process of determining maternity becomes particularly exposed in cases of partially or fully disembodied modes of reproduction. These create rough moments that can stall, hinder, or otherwise disrupt the smooth designation of maternity.

The two mix-up cases that I analyze below have similar stories on the surface: an embryo is transferred into the wrong patient, the mistake is discovered, and the dispute is taken to court. But they have quite different endings in terms of who is ultimately recognized as the authentic mother of the child in question, and whose family relationships and boundaries are protected or breached. I argue that maternity designation is an important yet overlooked sociolegal process in contemporary theorizing about motherhood and family. I define this designation as the activity of sorting through, affirming, or rejecting various maternal claims with the goal of assigning maternity to a specific person or persons. Viewing maternity as a designation or activity shifts the analytic lens from understanding maternity as a natural or definitive state to viewing it as the outcome of a sociolegal decision-making process. Parts of this process occur at the micro level via interpersonal interaction—for example, through identity work and negotiations between intended mothers and their surrogates or egg donors, the maternal claiming I described in the previous chapter based on prior research on surrogacy (Jacobson 2016; Teman 2010; Thompson 2005). However, the formal assignment of maternity typically occurs through meso-level organizations that interface with the state, such as hospitals and courts. I build on the notion of maternal claims making, by addressing it in these meso-level sites. Women might seek to assert maternal claims to a child, but that does not mean those claims will be formally recognized. Therefore, it is important to address both sides of this process: the claims making and the formal adjudication of such claims in court.

I identify four key sense-making tasks of the courts that are integral to their working through fragmented maternity:

recognizing diverse pathways to motherhood, clarifying conceptual boundaries of maternity, identifying legitimate (and illegitimate) bases of maternity, and affirming or denying maternal claims. Each of these tasks shows strong evidence of the contingent and uncertain nature of a maternity unmoored from its biological presumption. I use the concept of 'sense making' to indicate the interpretive process the courts go through when presented with the problem of maternity that does not fit neatly into prior definitions or customs. As Robert Lauer and Warren Handel (1977, 40) described in their discussion of symbolic interaction, "we are led to act by the stimulus of symbols. . . . [B]efore a response is made . . . that situation must be defined . . . the individual strives to make sense of it by representing it." Karl Weick (1995, 14–15) observed: "to engage in sensemaking is to construct, filter, frame, create facticity. . . . [This approaches] reality as an ongoing accomplishment that takes form when people make retrospective sense of situations in which they find themselves and their creations."

The two cases I analyze also introduce questions about inequality between the disputing parties. In the first case, the parental dispute was between two heterosexual married couples, one non-Hispanic white and the other Black. Given the historical devaluation of Black motherhood relative to white motherhood and the cultural pathologizing of the Black American family (Freeman 2020; Hill Collins 1990; D. Roberts 1997; Stacey 1996) we must not ignore the racial dynamics of the case. Although media coverage focused on the idea of a white woman giving birth to "black and white twins" (Arena 1999b), the court was largely silent on both the racial differences between the two potential mothers and the racial discordance between the white, gestational mother and the Black infant. I analyze this difference between the media fixation and legal silence to further understand how race might function, implicitly and explicitly, in designating maternity.

The second case pits a heterosexual married couple against a single woman. Perhaps surprisingly, the single woman retained her legal maternity as the birth mother, but the married man was granted legal paternity, visitation rights, and later split custody. As a result, two previously distinct family units were intertwined and their respective boundaries violated. Both women involved in the case were treated as having second-class familial relationships—the wife because she lacked a biological connection to the embryo that she and her husband intended to use, and the single woman because she had no male spouse to fill the role of presumed father of her child. Together, the two cases provide an opportunity to look at how courts are making sense of fragmented maternity and how this sense making occurs under conditions of family inequality.

Assisted Reproductive Technology Mix-Ups and Contested Maternity

Assisted reproductive technology mix-ups refer to any situation in which eggs, sperm, or embryos are mishandled outside of the body, resulting in the use of the wrong gametes or embryos during a reproductive procedure. Such mix-ups are rare but likely inevitable because assisted reproduction disembodies parts of the reproductive process, allowing opportunity for human error. Mix-ups are typically discovered when racial boundaries are crossed or when clinic staff members realize a labeling or clinical error has occurred after a procedure has taken place (Bender 2006; Mabry 2004). The first known U.S. case occurred in 1987, when a woman sought to use her husband's sperm posthumously to conceive a child (Mabry 2004). The child that she delivered had a notably darker skin tone than either she or her late husband, leading to the conclusion that the clinic had used the wrong sperm during insemination. While some of the mix-ups may lead patients to bring suit against clinics and physicians for such issues as wrongful birth or emotional harm (Fox 2019), others lead to situations of contested parentage. Embryos intended for one patient but placed into another create an unintentional fragmenting of maternity quite different from the intentional use of collaborative reproduction. Beyond the emotional and psychological implications, such cases potentially exist in legal limbo for at least two reasons. First, there is no clear documentation of intention and consent from the parties because the situation was not intended. Second, states use varying definitions of legal maternity in cases of IVF and collaborative reproduction (which I discuss more fully in chapter 6). Most states do not specifically address mixup scenarios and therefore must rely on more general legal principles or find analogous cases to address parentage disputes. Courts may also look to legislation that broadly governs collaborative reproductive practices in the state, even if specifics relevant to a given case are not available. Sometimes maternity cannot be contested once a woman has been established as the natural mother of a child (as happened in the second case, described below). Certain states continue to privilege the birth or gestational mother, while others favor intended parents in collaborative reproduction.

The 2017 Uniform Parentage Act (UPA) sought to address laboratory errors but only in the context of gestational surrogacy, basing its approach on a provision first passed as part of a UPA in Maine in 2015. Section 809(d) of the 2017 UPA reads (Uniform Law Commission (ULC) 2021c): "if, due to a clinical or laboratory error, a child conceived by assisted reproduction under a gestational surrogacy agreement is not genetically related to an intended parent or a donor who donated to the intended parent or parents, each intended parent, and not the gestational surrogate and the surrogate's spouse or former spouse, if any, is a parent of the child, subject to any other claim of parentage."

While this remedies the problem of creating potentially parentless children or leaving the gestational surrogate and her spouse on the hook for parentage, it makes little mention of the original providers of the reproductive cells other than to remark that final determinations are "subject to any other claim of parentage." As of this writing, three states have enacted the 2017 UPA or some variation of it, and either the act or a variation of it has been introduced in four other states. Adopting a variant of the UPA in 2018, Vermont addressed "laboratory errors" in assisted reproduction more generally, stating: "if due to a laboratory error the resulting child is not genetically related to either of the intended parents, the intended parents are the parents of the child unless otherwise determined by the court" (Vermont Statutes Annotated 2017). These approaches favor the unintended recipients of the embryo or gametes but also give substantial power to the courts to sort things out. After I analyze the two cases below, I offer some concluding thoughts on why approaches favoring the unintended recipient by default are likely to be harmful and unjust. Yet working out parental claims to mistakenly placed embryos also butts up against the politics of life. It is challenging to articulate moral and legal claims to an embryo or fetus without creating personhood along the way.

Case 1: Black and White Twins?

PERRY-ROGERS V. FASANO, 2000

In April 1998, two married women, Donna Fasano and Deborah Perry-Rogers, underwent embryo transfer procedures at a New York-based IVF clinic. Donna became pregnant with twins, but Deborah did not conceive. In May, two weeks into Donna's pregnancy, the IVF clinic informed both women that there had been a mistake. The embryologist had accidentally transferred both women's embryos into Donna's uterus. At the time, the clinic did not disclose to either woman who the other party was—likely due to concerns about violating medical privacy laws. After hearing this news, Donna sought DNA testing and discovered that one of the fetuses she was carrying was indeed not genetically related to her. Still, she opted to carry the pregnancy to term since both fetuses were healthy. In December 1998, Donna gave birth to two boys with very different skin tones, Vincent (white) and Joseph (Black). Donna and her husband were both non-Hispanic white. Deborah and her husband were both Black.

In March 1999, after learning from media reports that a white woman had given birth to "black and white twins" after an IVF mix-up, Deborah and her husband sued the Fasanos for custody of the Black infant and determination of parentage. After months of having no information about the whereabouts of their misplaced embryo, they assumed that Joseph was their genetic child. The next month, DNA tests affirmed this. In May 1999, nearly five months after the boys' birth, the Rogers were ultimately granted custody of Joseph, legally recognized as his parents, and allowed to revise his birth certificate to reflect them as the biological parents. They also later requested a legal name change, from Joseph Fasano to Akeil Rogers.

Not wanting to give up the baby completely, Donna Fasano requested visitation rights, chiefly on the grounds that the boys had bonded together in her womb and had been raised for the first few months of their lives as brothers. Although the Rogers were now confirmed as Joseph/Akeil's genetic parents, the custody agreement and transfer hinged on including the Fasanos' visitation rights. The Fasanos requested regular visits between the boys—visits that also required the Rogers to make the trip from their New Jersey home to Staten Island, where the Fasanos resided. This agreement also came with a hefty damages clause: the Rogers would have to pay $200,000 to the Fasanos if they reneged on visitation. Desperate to win custody of Joseph/Akeil, the Rogers initially agreed to visitation, which their attorney later noted was a decision made "under duress": "The Rogers have had to go through a hell of a lot here . . . [They] would have entered into an agreement in good faith that called on them to swim across the Hudson River to get their child back" (quoted in Wolfberg 1999).

Once Joseph/Akeil was securely in their custody, with legal documents affirming their parentage, the Rogers appealed to deny visitation. They argued that the Fasanos had no legal standing to request visitation, as New York domestic relations law restricted such rights to legal parents and blood-related siblings. In October 2000, two and a half years after the initial mix-up, the Rogers were granted exclusive parental rights to Joseph/Akeil. The court affirmed their parentage and denied the Fasanos' visitation rights, concluding: "where a child is properly in the custody of parents . . . [the parents have] broad rights to exclude any visitation, even by a person who has raised and nurtured the child as his or her own"

(*Perry-Rogers v. Fasano*, 2000). In response, the Fasanos quickly appealed, aiming to get Joseph/Akeil back in their custody. They asked for an evidentiary hearing on the 'best interests of the child', attempting to define the case now as a dispute between gestational and genetic mothers, even though they had already relinquished custody. This final attempt was met with a single statement from the court: "Motion for leave to appeal denied" (*Perry-Rogers v. Fasano*, 2001).

Some readers might feel that this story has a happy ending: the initial mix-up was resolved, and Joseph/Akeil made it back to his intended parents. The people originally intending to use the embryo for family building were granted custody and then exclusive parental rights to the child born from that embryo. However, other readers may feel that the ending robbed the Fasanos of a child that Donna had gestated, birthed, and raised along with his twin, Vincent, for the first five months of his life. In any case, it took two and a half years to legally resolve the issues that the mix-up created. This lengthy period from mistake to ultimate resolution clearly reflects legal uncertainty over post-IVF forms of maternity and kinship. For instance, does gestation warrant maternity in the absence of both a genetic connection and the intention to become a parent to that specific child? What does it mean, legally and culturally, for fetuses to share in utero space but not be genetically related?

Figure 5.1 diagrams the connections between the parties in the case. There was no question that the Fasanos were the biological and legal parents of Vincent (the white infant). He was conceived from their conjugal embryo, and Donna Fasano had gestated and given birth to him: her maternal connection to him was fully integrated. The use of IVF aside, Richard, Donna, and Vincent Fasano fit within the framework of the repronormative family. Deborah Perry-Rogers and Robert Rogers had used their own conjugal embryo to create Joseph/Akeil. However, the IVF mix-up unintentionally fragmented Deborah's maternity: Donna Fasano ended up gestating and giving birth to Joseph/Akeil. In light of this, the court was confronted with thinking through inadvertently created relationships.

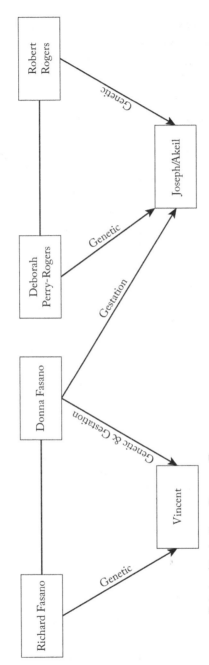

FIG. 5.1. Relationships in *Perry-Rogers v. Fasano*

In chapter 4, I described how forms of post-IVF maternity are highly contingent. They rely on different factors that come together to make maternity intelligible (especially to potential users of collaborative reproduction who might be anxious about losing fully integrated biological maternity). But how do fragmented and contingent maternal claims hold up under legal scrutiny? Donna Fasano initially justified having visitation and her potential maternity rights through her bond with Joseph/Akeil during and after pregnancy, as well as the bond between the two boys—which had developed out of sharing one womb for nine months and then being raised together for five months after birth. Although gestation can be defined as a biological relationship, Donna emphasized the psychological and social aspects of in utero bonding as well as five months of parenting after birth. Notably, in cases of intentional gestational surrogacy, physicians have often argued that the lack of genetic connection between surrogate and fetus should decrease the "risk of bonding to the pregnancy" (Leeton 2013, 76). However, this view clearly creates problems for thinking about maternal bonding in egg donation, which fully severs maternal genetics. And arguably the idea of not bonding to a pregnancy simply because you lack a genetic relationship largely functions symbolically. For intentional surrogates, lacking such a tie reinforces that the surrogate is not an expectant mother of the child-to-be (Berend 2016; Teman 2010). Of course, Donna Fasano was also carrying a mixed genetic pregnancy. Is it possible to bond with only one fetus in a multiple pregnancy?

In chapter 4, I also emphasized the importance of the conjugal embryo in solidifying fragmented and contingent maternal claims. Yet even though Joseph/Akeil was conceived from the Rogers's conjugal embryo, it was Donna Fasano who had control over the decision of whether to give him to his genetic parents. According to media coverage of the case, "lawyers agree that the woman who gives birth is legally considered the child's mother regardless of DNA" (Gross and Harpaz 1999). Surrogacy at that time was prohibited by New York law (New York Domestic Relations Law 2021), with surrogacy contracts considered "contrary to the public policy of this state . . . void and unenforceable." Therefore, no law explicitly addressed situations of genetic-only maternity at the time of this parentage conflict. Precedent set by a New York egg donation case just a few years before decidedly favored Deborah Perry-Rogers's maternal claims over Donna's. In *McDonald v. McDonald* (1994),[1] the Supreme Court of the State of New York relied on the test of procreative intent, which was developed in the landmark California case of *Johnson v. Calvert* (1993). Where there is a "tie" for maternity between a genetic and a gestational mother, intent is considered more foundational because the more natural mother is the one intending from the beginning to conceive and raise the child. Deborah possessed the procreative intent to conceive a child with that specific embryo, and by that logic she, not Donna, was the original and more authentic mother of that child. Nonetheless, *Perry-Rogers v. Fasano* (2000) was not so neatly decided at the outset.

Because of general legal ambiguity concerning collaborative reproduction at that time and the weight of legal tradition favoring birth mothers, the Rogers could not compel Donna Fasano to turn over their genetic child to them. Instead, they had to wait for Donna to decide to do so. Holding this legal power, Donna asserted that she and her family had some rights to continued contact with the child. The initial custody decision and several subsequent appeals favored the notion that the boys had a relationship that was worthy of legal protection and preservation. The relationship between Vincent and Joseph/Akeil can be viewed as a twist on fraternal twinship: two eggs that came from two different genetic sources. Culturally, the twin relationship is often viewed "with a sense of wonder and awe" (Fraley and Tancredy 2012, 308).[2] At the same time, the boys' twin relationship was a by-product of a medical mix-up. Were they truly twins? Experts offered different interpretations of the situation. For instance, an article in the Associated Press (Gross and Harpaz 1999) first quotes George Annas, a professor of health law at Boston University, as saying "they are twins, raised in the same uterus. They've been together for 14 months [including gestation]. They're twins in every sense—except genetic." The article later quotes Sean Tipton, speaking on behalf of the ASRM, who commented: "this is a pretty clear-cut mistake."

After custody had been transferred to the Rogers and the Fasanos' visitation rights paused and awaiting clarification, the court had to work through the different maternal and other relational or kinship claims presented. The court observed that the Fasanos had implicitly recognized Deborah Perry-Rogers and her husband as Joseph/Akeil's rightful parents when the Fasanos had voluntarily ceded custody. As Deborah had not given birth, her maternal claim was primarily through her genetic relationship, but the court noted that this was also supported by her and her husband's procreative intent: "It was they [Deborah and her husband] who purposefully arranged for their genetic material to be taken . . . to create their own child . . . whom they intended to rear" (as quoted in *Perry-Rogers v. Fasano* 2000). In aiming to void the Fasanos' visitation rights, the Rogers' lawyer argued that Donna and Vincent Fasano were "genetic strangers" to Joseph/Akeil and therefore had no legal standing to seek visitation. The court agreed that Donna was a "genetic stranger" to Joseph/Akeil, but it did not deny her maternity purely on that basis, anticipating that doing so could set a precedent for defining maternity solely as a genetic relationship. Instead, the court relied on what it viewed as more fundamental to the situation: the embryo had been mistakenly implanted, and the Fasanos knew about the mistake almost immediately after conception: "[the Fasanos'] nominal parenthood should have been treated as a mistake to be corrected as soon as possible, before development of a parental relationship" (as quoted in *Perry-Rogers v. Fasano* 2000).

While the court affirmed that bonding between a gestational mother and child "before, during, and after birth," as well as potentially between infants who were together in the womb, was a legitimate issue to be considered, "the suggested existence of a bond is not enough under the present circumstances." It further reasoned: "any bonding on the part of Akeil to his gestational mother and her family was the direct result of the Fasanos' failure to take timely action upon being informed [of the mistake]." The court declared that Donna Fasano was attempting to base her maternity on an illegitimate foundation (i.e., a mistake). The court opined that the situation was more analogous to one in which infants had been switched at birth than to a dispute between genetic and gestational mothers.

The analogy of being 'switched at birth' could offer a useful model for sorting out IVF mix-ups. Yet the court's discussion of the mistake needing to be corrected and the Fasanos' "failure to take timely action" raises some concerns. For instance, what timely action might the Fasanos have taken once they learned about the mix-up? One option would be to pursue selective reduction, which refers to selective termination of one (or more) fetuses in a multiple pregnancy. But this comes with its own set of risks, such as higher rates of preterm birth and the risk of a procedure-related loss of a desired fetus. Therefore, selective reduction has typically been used only to reduce higher-order multiples (triplets and above) down to twin pregnancies to decrease pregnancy complications and improve health outcomes (Dodd and Crowther 2004; Wimalasundera 2010). Additionally, selectively terminating a fetus might resolve the problem of having a fetus inside the wrong uterus, but it would not resolve the involuntary childlessness of the other couple. The Rogers would have paid for the IVF cycle and then had their genetic fetus terminated. This idea of the Fasanos failing to take action also obscures the responsibility of the fertility clinic and practitioners, who were ultimately the actors who made the mistake. The "failure to take timely action" might also refer to the post birth period when the Fasanos did not attempt to communicate with or locate the genetic progenitors of the embryo that produced Joseph/Akeil. Yet what should or could they have done in light of the clinic's not providing information about the parties to one another?

Case 2: Mom, Son, Dad, and?

ROBERT B. V. SUSAN B., 2003

In June 2000, a heterosexual married couple, Robert and Denise B., went to a California fertility clinic. Denise underwent embryo transfer using an embryo created with a donated egg and Robert's sperm. She became pregnant and gave birth to a girl, Madeline, in February 2001. The couple then froze their excess embryos for later use. Also in February 2001, Susan, a single woman in her late forties, gave birth to a baby boy, Daniel. Susan had gone to the same fertility clinic as Robert and Denise for her embryo transfer procedure, seeking to use embryos that she had created from anonymous egg and sperm donors. Coincidentally, both Denise and Susan had selected the same egg donor, which may have contributed to the mix-up that followed. Ten months after the births of the babies, Robert, Denise, and Susan found out that there had been a mistake—three of Denise and Robert's embryos had been implanted in Susan's uterus. None of Susan's embryos had been used. Denise and Robert immediately sought contact with baby Daniel. When Susan refused to turn over custody to them, they brought a parentage action against her.

Figure 5.2 shows the relationships in *Robert B. v. Susan B.* Unlike in *Perry-Rogers v. Fasano* (2000), none of the parties here knew of the mistake until after the babies were born. Indeed, they did not find out until nineteen months after the original embryo transfer, when the babies were around ten months old. Susan gave birth to and nurtured Daniel under the assumption that he was her rightful child through collaborative reproduction. She had never intended to use her own eggs, so she never expected a genetic maternal connection.

Another crucial difference between the two cases was that the embryo that became Daniel was genetically related to Robert but not Denise. In that sense, it was not a true conjugal embryo, containing genetic material from both of them. These differences contextualize the different outcome of the two cases. The court ultimately defined Robert (the husband and sperm provider) as Daniel's "natural father" and Susan (the single woman who gave birth to and raised the baby) as his natural mother. As for Robert's wife, Denise, who was the legal mother of Daniel's full genetic sibling, the court ruled that she had provided "no [solid] basis for either challenging Susan's maternity status or establishing her own" (quoted in *Robert B. v. Susan B.* 2003). Susan was awarded

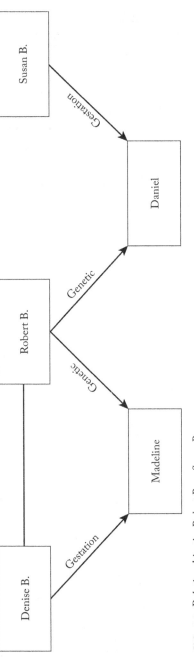

FIG. 5.2. Relationships in *Robert B. v. Susan B.*

temporary full custody of Daniel, while Robert was first given weekly visitation rights and later awarded split custody (Bender 2006).[3] How did the court determine parentage?

Susan's maternal claims were rooted in being Daniel's gestational mother as well as in the fact that she had raised and nurtured him as her child for ten months after birth: she was informed of the embryo mix-up only after nineteen months of gestation, birth, and mothering. The court also recognized Susan's intent to receive "genetic material from 'two strangers'" (quoted in *Robert B. v. Susan B.* 2003): the anonymous donors she had selected to create her embryos. In an effort to protect the integrity of her family unit, Susan tried to establish that Robert should be treated as a sperm donor. If Robert's legal paternity could not be established, this might also weaken Denise's maternal claims, because Denise had no type of biological tie to Daniel.

However, the Court did not agree to define Robert as a donor. Under California law, a donor is someone who explicitly intends to provide gametes for a person other than their reproductive partner (California Family Code 2020). Testing affirmed Robert's biological paternity, but it was his intentions that solidified his claim. He had intended that his sperm be used to contribute to an embryo that his wife would gestate and that they would raise the subsequent child together. What about Denise? At the time of this case, only cisgendered men could benefit from the indirect logic of the marital presumption—women could not argue that they had a maternal relationship to a child based on their marital relationship to that child's biological father.[4] However, Denise's lawyer argued that Denise theoretically "stood in the shoes of a genetic mother" (quoted in *Robert B. v. Susan B.* 2003) because the anonymous egg donor had transferred her genetic parental rights to Denise via the donation agreement signed at the fertility clinic. While the court recognized that Denise had contractual rights to the embryos and established that the embryos technically belonged to Robert and Denise, such rights could not be conflated with parentage. To do so, the court noted, would reflect parentage as a form of ownership over a child: "Any contractual rights Denise had to the embryos . . . but now what we're talking about is a live person, not an embryo" (quoted in *Robert B. v. Susan B.* 2003). Denise also tried to delegitimize Susan's maternity by asking the court for an opportunity to show that "Susan colluded with the fertility clinic to obtain the embryo" (quoted in *Robert B. v. Susan B.* 2003). However, there was no evidence that any collusion had occurred—the mix-up simply resulted from an unfortunate error by the clinic.

Denise's maternal claims were not rejected solely because she lacked a biological connection to Daniel. The court recognized that a woman does not need to have a biological relationship to a child to "determine the existence or non-existence of a mother and child relationship [under the Uniform Parentage Act]" (quoted in *Robert B. v. Susan B.* 2003). Yet the court also noted that Susan had already "clearly established a mother-child relationship by the undisputed fact that she gave birth to Daniel." Therefore, Denise could not now seek to establish her own maternity: "California law recognizes only one natural mother." Susan had simply claimed the spot first.

Although maternity did not require a biological foundation, the court also found that procreative intent in the absence of any biological ties was an insufficient maternal claim. Referring to *Johnson v. Calvert* (1993), the court noted: "The concept of 'intended mother' is employed as a tiebreaker only when two women have equal claims by 'genetic consanguinity' and childbirth" (quoted in *Robert B. v. Susan B.* 2003). But the court also recognized that procreative intent was somewhat muddled here: "Susan intended to be the mother of a child created from an embryo . . . but not *that* embryo. . . . Denise intended to be the mother of the child created from this very embryo . . . but not at that time [it had been frozen for later use] and she did not intend for another woman to bear the child" (*Robert B. v. Susan B.* 2003). Although Susan was lacking clear intent, she had given birth and already started to raise baby Daniel; therefore, the court chose to uphold Susan's more natural maternity over Denise's.

Table 5.1 summarizes the maternal claims made by or on behalf of each woman in the two embryo mix-up cases. These claims did not flow from singular sources, nor were they consistently deployed across the two cases. Indeed, given these different outcomes in the cases and the multiple bases for asserting maternal claims, how can we sort out post-IVF forms of maternity?

Both courts were faced with the task of recognizing diverse pathways to maternity as a function of postmodern family building in the post-IVF era. Indeed, this was a primary consideration for the courts to agree to hear these cases as opposed to simply relying on the legal tradition of the presumption of biology. In recognizing diverse pathways to motherhood—gestation, genetics, bonding or nurturing, procreative intent, and so on—the courts also explicitly expanded the historical legal concept of maternity to encompass various possibilities. For instance, in *Perry-Rogers v. Fasano* (2000), the court observed: "Given the complex possibilities . . . it is simply inappropriate to render any determination solely as a consequence of genetics. It is certainly conceivable that under some other circumstances, we would have to treat both genetic and gestational mother[s] as parents." Referring to the California Uniform Parentage Act, which contained parentage provisions for assisted reproduction, the court in *Robert B. and Denise B. v. Susan B.* (2003) similarly noted: "On its face, this provision does not restrict . . . alleged mothers to those who are genetically or gestationally related to the child."

Yet even as they formally recognized that women could become mothers in diverse ways, the courts also worked to identify the conceptual boundaries of maternity. That is, before they could adequately weigh the different arguments presented, they had to clarify what maternity might consist of. Maternity could not be a free-for-all status. For instance, both courts asserted that there was only one natural mother of a child who could be legally recognized. In doing so, they defined maternity as a relationship that exists

TABLE 5.1 Maternal Claims and Final Designations

	BASIS FOR MATERNAL CLAIM						
	GESTATION	GENETICS	MOTHERING	RIGHTS[a]	RELATIONSHIP WITH BIOLOGICAL FATHER	MOTHER OF SIBLING	PROCREATIVE INTENT
Perry-Rogers v. Fasano							
Donna Fasano	x		x	x		x[b]	
Deborah Rogers		x		x	x		x
Robert B. v. Susan B.							
Denise B.		x[c]		x	x	x	x
Susan B.	x		x	x			x

NOTES: Shaded rows indicate maternal designations by the courts. [a] Rights include both those that were specifically recognized by the court (such as the right to custody) and those that were presumed (such as the right to create a reproductive contract). [b] The relationship of mother of sibling was not recognized by the court. [c] Denise argued she stood in the place of the genetic mother by using a donor egg.

between one woman and her child or children. This logic would exclude any additional parties from claiming maternity (or a maternal-like relationship) once that role was officially filled. For example, in *Perry-Rogers v. Fasano* (2000), the court declared that once a child was in parental custody, the legal parents could deny visitation by other parties—"even by a person who has raised and nurtured the child as his or her own." Therefore, raising and nurturing a child, while important evidence of de facto parenting on its own (Nejaime 2021), could not sufficiently constitute maternity if there was already a legally recognized mother to a child. Additionally, in *Robert B. and Denise B. v. Susan B.* (2003), the court observed that "two appellate courts . . . have refused to recognize a biologically *unrelated* woman as an 'interested person'" for adjudicating maternity. Without some type of biological connection (e.g., eggs or gestation), the court saw little basis for establishing maternity, even if the relevant party had other elements of a maternal-like relationship, such as procreative intent.

The courts also had to identify il/legitimate bases on which women might found their maternal claims. The court recognized that many of Donna Fasano's claims were quite legitimate on the surface: such as being the gestational mother and bonding pre- and postnatally to baby Joseph/Akeil. But it identified the ultimate base of those claims—the "'mistake' that was not immediately corrected" (quoted in *Perry-Rogers v. Fasano* 2000)—as illegitimate. According to the court, Donna might have had some of the relevant qualities of legal maternity in regard to Joseph/Akeil, but she did not have the original or authentic right to claim that status. In contrast, Susan B.'s very similar maternal claims to Daniel (gestation and a nurturance or care relationship after birth), were considered legitimate, but only because she did not know about the clinic's error. Although Denise B. claimed that Susan had "colluded" with the clinic to gain access to its embryos, the court determined that she lacked appropriate evidence of that collusion. If such evidence had existed, it might have made Susan's maternity illegitimate, as having been established under false pretense. In addressing the foundations of Denise's maternal claims, the court acknowledged that while she might have had certain contractual rights to the embryos, those rights did not extend to Daniel. Contractual rights were not legitimate foundations for parent-child relationships. After working through the logic of each of the above tasks, the courts not only had to affirm those maternal claims that were supported and deemed legitimate, but they also had to deny any maternal claims that were deemed insufficient or illegitimate.

Unequal Maternities?

The two cases above also raise questions about race, marital status, and motherhood. Media coverage of *Perry-Rogers v. Fasano* emphasized the idea of a white woman giving birth to "black and white twins." Yet the court was largely silent on race as a factor in sorting out maternity, appearing to take a color-blind approach. In the final published opinion, the court made only two references to race, first noting that the boys were of "two different races" then stating that Vincent was a "white child" and Joseph/Akeil was a "black child." Beyond this, race was perhaps peculiarly absent from any discussion of parentage. However, there were frequent references to "blood," "biology," and "genetics." These are terms have often been used to refer to race, especially racial classification via the so-called "one drop" rule (Gotanda 1995; K. Eyer 2014). Yet my reading here is that the terms referred more specifically to the types of biological connections that the different women had to the infant. Thus, their usage in this context was seemingly devoid of racial connotations. Furthermore, the court did not rely on racial concordance as a guiding doctrine to reunite the Black genetic family or on racial discordance to deny the white woman's maternal claims to Joseph/Akeil. This is somewhat surprising, given the long history of explicit race-matching policies in family law for adoption or fostering cases (K. Eyer 2014) and the cultural conception that "the (heterosexual) family is . . . a site of gender difference . . . [and] racial sameness" (Russell 2018, 28). But as the philosopher Camisha Russell (2018, 23) reminds us, "race seems always to be lurking just below the surface when it comes to assisted reproduction." A color-blind legal approach is predicated on the assumption that parties have an "equal starting point," which ignores the historical subordination of Blackness and "the cumulative disadvantages that are the starting point for so many black citizens" (Gotanda 1995, 266). Whiteness is a privileged racial status, especially in the context of the repronormative family. The racial politics here are thrown in sharp relief when we ask: How might things have gone differently if the mistaken embryo had been implanted into the Black mother's uterus? Would Deborah Perry-Rogers have felt entitled to argue that she had a right to a child created from a white couple's conjugal embryo? Would her claims to a white infant and her assertions of kinship between the boys have been so easily validated by the court? Would she have been granted visitation rights?

Research on transracial surrogacy provides some insight here.[5] Most often when there are racial differences between a gestational surrogate and the intended parents, the surrogate is a woman of color, while the intended parents are white (Harrison 2016). Often this difference is further compounded by social class differences, given the relative cost of assisted reproduction in the United States and abroad. Race is constructed as an essential characteristic of the gametes and embryos, thereby infused in genetics (Deomampo 2019). In contrast, surrogate wombs are largely race neutral—at least in terms of influencing the racial categorization of the child-to-be. Racial discordance between a nonwhite surrogate and a white child-to-be can be strategic: it serves to recast the surrogate as providing care for, but not being the authentic mother of, the child-to-be (Harrison 2016; Thompson 2005).

Many scholars would point to *Johnson v. Calvert* as instructive here, although it is not a true counterfactual to *Perry-Rogers v. Fasano*. Anna Johnson, a Black gestational surrogate, sought to assert her maternal claims to the baby she was carrying for the Calverts, a married, heterosexual couple. Mark Calvert was white, and Christina Calvert was Filipina. It was their conjugal embryo that Anna agreed to gestate on their behalf. This case caused a stir not simply because Anna lacked a genetic connection to the baby she was carrying, but also because of the racial discordance between surrogate and child. As the legal scholar Anita Allen (1991, 19) remarked, "for the first time in history, an African-American woman had given birth to a child exclusively of European and Philippine ancestry." The eventual outcome of *Johnson v. Calvert*[6] created the legal test of 'procreative intent' to use when there was a tie between gestational and genetic mothers. But this language of having a tie between two equally situated mothers is rather superficial. Is it really a tie when a heterosexual married couple of privileged race and class status are competing for parentage against a Black single mother?[7] Would it have been a tie if Donna Fasano and Deborah Perry-Rogers were battling over the maternity of a white infant? It seems more likely that the court would have used a legal test that swiftly placed the white infant in exclusive custody of the white parents.

Beyond the racial politics of collaborative reproduction, we also have to recognize the long and fraught history of Black women's relationships to white children. Relations of care between Black women and white children have not necessarily created legitimate maternal claims to those children. The controlling image of the Black mammy as the "faithful, obedient domestic servant" created a situation in which enslaved Black women were intimately involved with white families but remained subordinate to "elite, white male power" (Hill Collins 1990, 71). A variation of this relationship has continued under more contemporary conditions of "diverted mothering" (Wong 1994), in which Black women have continued to raise and care for children of white families without being legitimately part of those families. Allen (1991, 23) aptly noted: "I suspect that few regard Black women as the appropriate legal mothers of children who are not at least part Black. Blacks are not supposed to have [or want] white children." By contrast, whiteness has long made it possible to legitimately claim nonwhite children, often framed as 'saving' Black and brown children through transracial adoption and fostering practices (Jennings 2006). Furthermore, white middle-class motherhood is elevated as sacred and ideal, through the cult of true womanhood and domesticity (Hays 1996), and juxtaposed with the cultural ideology of the deviant, irresponsible, and degenerate motherhood of Black women (Freeman 2020; Hill Collins 1990; D. Roberts 1997). Thus, white mothers and white families have historically had privileged access to both white and nonwhite children. One caveat here is that white women who give birth to biracial children in the context of an interracial relationship are often viewed as "crossing social boundaries" (Verbian 2006, 213), challenging ideologies of family and kinship that expect biological family members to have the same racial categorization.

Yet it was the privileged cultural status of the white mother that distinctly came through in the media coverage of *Perry-Rogers v. Fasano* (2000).[8] The media focused on the maternal claims and emotions of the white woman as a distraught mother and paid minimal attention to the loss and grief experienced by the Black mother, who was desperately seeking her child. In a statement to the press, Donna Fasano's lawyer described her decision to give Joseph/Akeil to the Rogers as "heart-wrenching" and "an ultimate act of love" after much "soul-searching" and agonizing over the situation: "She loves her boys . . . she doesn't look at them as black and white. She looks at them as her sons. She is torn apart by this" (quoted in *Advance Staff Report* 1999). Similarly, in June, after the custody transfer, the Fasanos' lawyer stated: "They wanted to fight to keep Joseph in the beginning. . . . In her heart, Mrs. Fasano feels she is the mother and her husband is the father. It was very hard to do this, but in the long run they felt it was best for the child." (quoted in Arena 1999a). The emphasis on Donna's maternal love for both children invites the reader to sympathize with and culturally authenticate her maternal claim to both boys. She feels "in her heart" that they are "her sons." Her maternal love is also described as unconditional and specifically colorblind: "she doesn't look at them as black and white." And while the reader does not have any idea of what Donna was actually thinking or feeling, we are invited to imagine the depth of her maternal emotions.

Additionally, much of the coverage before the custody transfer described Donna Fasano as deciding to "surrender," "give up," or "turn over" Joseph/Akeil to the Rogers. This conjures up the image of a birth mother giving up her child to waiting, adoptive parents, and the ensuing emotions. These terms also contrast with the language deployed by many intentional gestational surrogates (Jacobson 2016; Teman 2010), as well as the unintentional surrogate mother in the Savage-Morell mix-up case—in which the Carolyn Savage referred to giving back "someone else's child" (quoted in Anonymous 2009). Some of this differential coverage of the two mothers may have been a result of the different strategies advised by the couples' legal teams. Indeed, some reports referred to the Fasanos heading out to meet with the press, while the Rogers left through the back door, shying away from publicity. Yet we also cannot ignore how the media depicted Donna's emotions and heartbreak—emphasizing her maternal love and sacrifice—at the expense of Deborah Perry-Roger's experience of being deprived of maternity.

In February 2020, two decades later, an article in the *Australian Women's Weekly* (Gannon 2020) covering IVF mix-ups continued to frame the case as one in which the white mother and her family made the ultimate sacrifice: "On May 10, 1999, when the babies were five months old, Donna and Richard separated their twins, said a tearful goodbye to Joseph, and handed him over to two strangers." Depicting the Rogers as "two strangers" invokes them as outsiders, nonfamily, who were taking a child away from the distraught parents, as opposed to focusing on a reunion between parents and a desperately sought-after child, or on the emotional distress that both families faced because of the mix-up. I think that the media coverage would have been quite different if the embryo creating Vincent, the white infant, had accidentally been placed in Deborah's uterus.

While race was the major distinction between the disputing mothers in *Perry-Rogers v. Fasano*, the second case pitted a heterosexual married couple against a single mother in claiming parentage of Daniel. Intriguingly, this case ended with Denise, the single mother, having her legal maternity affirmed as she was declared to be the natural mother of Daniel. Yet this case raises questions about both marital status and biology in legitimating maternal claims. Both Susan and Denise had second-class familial claims in relation to Daniel. Susan lacked a male spouse to fill the presumptive paternal role, and Denise lacked a biological tie to challenge Susan's natural maternity. This case seems much less tidy than *Perry-Rogers v. Fasano*, because it did not involve a true conjugal embryo and because both families gestated, birthed, and raised children for a more extended period of time before they knew anything about the mix-up.

Following the procreative intent test, Denise should have been awarded parentage—but we cannot and should not ignore the gestational and social maternal connections that Susan had to Daniel. This case challenges us to understand how complicated disembodied reproductive practices can be in thinking about maternity. There seems to be no right decision that would undo much of the harm of the initial mix-up, mostly because of how long it was concealed from the parties. Denise should have had a recognized right to the embryos she created with her spouse: their plans to have a future baby together with the misplaced embryo were foiled, and they were deprived of their exclusive parentage of Daniel. The gendered asymmetry of parentage overtly comes through here in the fact that Robert could make a parentage claim to baby Daniel, but Denise ultimately could not (Bender 2006). Would the outcome have been different if Denise had used her own egg in conjunction with her husband's sperm, thus creating a true conjugal embryo from their combined genetic material? An analysis based on procreative intent would have given more weight to recognizing Denise's maternal claims to Daniel, but ultimately her maternity was considered less than authentic in the hierarchy of motherhood (Letherby 1999). If everything had gone according to plan and the embryo had made it securely into Denise's body instead of Susan's, Denise's maternity would have been unquestioned. But her lack of any biological tie demoted her to a legal stranger—something of a paradox, since she was considered the birth and legal mother of Daniel's full genetic sibling.

But Susan was also deprived in this scenario, even though her maternity was legally affirmed. She was denied exclusive parentage in relation to Daniel, the baby she had gestated, birthed, and raised intentionally on her own for ten months before learning about the mistake. It is possible that the outcome would have been different if Susan had had a male spouse to claim the spot of a presumptive father for Daniel. With her biolegal maternity secure, the case might have hinged on determining whether biological or social paternity was more important and might have used a 'best interests of the child' test to not disturb an intact (read: complete with two parents) family.[9] Both Denise's and Susan's maternal claims, then, were viewed by the court as missing crucial elements to be considered sufficient on their own. This is a particular characteristic of fragmented maternity: its contingent nature leaves it open to scrutiny and to being socially and legally discredited.

Unintended Parents

Cases involving IVF mix-ups and contested maternity highlight the risk and uncertainty of postmodern family building through assisted and collaborative reproduction. They also show how much we need a comprehensive and consistent regulatory framework to sort out parentage and minimize harm to individuals and families. Although feminist scholarship has noted the primacy of genetics in U.S. culture (Ragone 1999; Rothman 1989), the human egg does not emerge as the fundamental basis of maternity in either of the cases analyzed in this chapter. A variety of claims are brought under consideration by courts, but none are truly given primacy to set clear rules for defining maternity. Rather, a constellation of factors related to each scenario is taken into consideration to arrive at the ultimate designation of maternity. In both cases, there is an attempt to simultaneously broaden as well as limit the definition of maternity through the court's decision-making process. Ultimately, however, there is no new or replacement theory of maternity that rises to the top when maternity is biologically fragmented. Additionally, maternity designation, in the absence of clear legal frameworks, leaves a substantial amount of discretion to the courts.

While regulatory gaps are one of the problems plaguing assisted and collaborative reproduction in the United States, the simple presence of regulation is not always positive (see chapter 6). The current approach of the 2017 Uniform Parentage Act to laboratory errors favors the unintended recipients of misplaced reproductive cells. But reproductive cells and parent-child relationships are not fungible. Intended parents are looking to become not a parent in general, but a parent to a child from a particular embryo. People invest their desires, emotions, and resources in achieving pregnancy with either cells from their own bodies or those from carefully chosen donors and surrogates. Expectant parenthood is a particular social, emotional, and legal status oriented toward the child-to-be. Treating it as anything less is to treat it as a second-class form of parenthood. Favoring the parental claims of unintended recipients who accidentally receive someone else's reproductive cells has the potential to create significant harm and injustice. At the same time, I do not think that the best solution in all scenarios is to ignore or invalidate the parental claims of unintended recipients. We need to recognize the pain of all parties involved in these mix-ups and work out humane solutions to the extent that they are possible. There are several questions about how to best do this. Should people unintentionally involved in the creation of a child have recourse to visitation or a right to custody? What would this mean for the exclusive rights of parentage that grant parents "a fundamental right to the control, care, and custody of their children" (Cahn 2009, 27)?

One answer, of course, is to create stricter standards in clinics to minimize potential mix-ups and to have well-defined protocols in place for notifying patients immediately if a mistake occurs. This likely would have facilitated an easier solution to the second case discussed above, as a major difference between it and the first case was the fact that none of the parties in the second case knew about the mix-up until months after the baby involved was born. The ASRM Ethics Committee officially weighed in on medical errors involving reproductive cells, noting that IVF clinics have a "duty to disclose" errors out of respect for patient autonomy (2006b,

513; 2011, 1312; and 2016, 59). The committee noted that in cases where errors might lead to "unintended genetic parentage," clinics have obligations to inform patients "without exception. . . . [T]he patient's right to know is compelling" (2006b, 513). This outlines standards for disclosure and underscores the urgency of unintended parentage from mix-ups, but it does little to resolve the implications of medical errors after they occur.

Another answer here is to rely on the analogy that the court used in *Perry-Rogers v. Fasano*, likening the situation to a case of newborns being switched at birth. Although there were some problems with this, as I noted above, this analogy serves to highlight the particulars of parenthood: you do not just expect to leave the hospital with any infant, you expect to leave with your infant. Similarly, you do not expect to leave an IVF clinic implanted with any embryo, you expect to have received your embryo (whether biological or chosen). Combined with the test of procreative intent, the analogy of switched at birth could offer some clarity in sorting out IVF mistakes. Additionally, the switched at birth analogy is not a deterministic directive to return children to a particular set of parents. It also relies on the factors of the specific situation and the best interests of the child (Foote 1999). Other possible analogies here include cases of unintended pregnancy, in which the biological parents never had or do not wish to continue a relationship with one another; co-parenting arrangements resulting from relationship dissolutions; and adoption (Miller 2010).

But using several of the above analogies could create a slippery slope for embryonic and fetal personhood: the fundamental issue to be corrected regarded not full-fledged humans but switched reproductive cells. Thus, a major recurring issue here is how to recognize rights to embryos that function as parental rights without granting embryos a legal status (Cromer 2019; Miller 2010). The politics of life continues to rear its head in scenarios that do not overtly address abortion. However, abortion does directly enter the equation when we think about unintended parentage and the right to terminate a pregnancy from a mix-up. Regardless of the rights that other people may have to the embryos, women should not become unwitting surrogates: they should not be obliged to have babies for someone else. Carolyn Savage made the choice to continue her pregnancy as a surrogate, but the conditions of her unwitting surrogacy also led to her ensuing psychological and emotional distress. Nor should women be compelled to terminate pregnancies, especially if there are multiple embryos that were destined to have multiple intended parents (as in the first case analyzed above). Women who become pregnant, whether for their own families or for other families, must retain their full reproductive rights and autonomy. Thus, we need to consider the entire constellation of potentially colliding rights in these unintentional collaborative scenarios.

6

Adopting or Resisting
New Maternities?

It has now been four decades since the first IVF baby was born in the United States, and nearly as long since the country's first successful egg donation and gestational surrogacy pregnancies. The most recent reports from the CDC (2022) show that assisted and collaborative forms of reproduction currently account for around 2 percent of all US births. In 2019, the latest year for which full national data are available, this amounted to 83,946 babies. Assisted and collaborative reproduction is firmly part of the reality of postmodern family building. However, currently fewer than half of the states have either statutory or case law explicitly addressing maternity in collaborative reproduction. This is not because of a lack of guidance or awareness of the issues. Since the late nineteenth century, the Uniform Law Commission (ULC) has led deliberations on and drafted uniform and model acts to assist state lawmaking activities.[1] In 1973, the ULC drafted the first Uniform Parentage Act (UPA) for states to adopt (ULC 2021a). The goal of the 1973 UPA was to eliminate legal distinctions between legitimate and illegitimate children and ensure clearly defined paths to paternity for all children. The act also addressed paternity via AID, to guarantee the legal status of AID-conceived children. This was followed by a 1988 model act addressing IVF and traditional surrogacy, called the Uniform Status of Children of Assisted Conception

Act. In 2000 and 2017, the ULC updated the UPA, in part to account for the growing use of collaborative reproduction (ULC 2021b and 2021c). Still, only a minority of U.S. states have adopted any form of the UPA, either in full or in part (Table 6.1). Of course, states can draft their own statutes rather than adopting the ULC's model legislation, and several have chosen to do so.

In this chapter I focus on state lawmaking regarding collaborative reproduction. First, I briefly look at states' statutory laws to get a sense of the number and timing of states that have adopted parentage laws regarding collaborative reproduction. Then, I conduct an in-depth case analysis of Louisiana statutes on IVF and collaborative reproduction for the period 1986–2016. I use these two different approaches to provide both an overall sketch of state-level variation in regulating collaborative reproduction and a closer view of sense-making activities during the legislative process.

I focus on Louisiana because of both its potential distinctiveness and its typicality as a case of interest. In terms of distinctiveness, Louisiana was the first state to enact statutory law addressing IVF and parentage through embryo donation. But it also did not adopt any version of the UPA, instead employing a rather piecemeal approach to regulating assisted and collaborative reproduction over the next thirty years. This at times leads to contradictory ideas about what qualifies as legal maternity, a point I discuss more fully below. I also view Louisiana as a potentially typical case in terms of its geographic location in the American South and its political history as a "ruby red" state (Bridges 2020; see also Cahn and Carbone 2010). Substantial attention has been paid to "mega states" on the East and West Coasts, such as New York and California (Markens 2007, 2; see also Heidt-Forsythe 2018), since these states are seen as drivers of public discourse and policy making because of their population size and relative concentration of fertility industry activities (Spar 2006). In contrast, southern states have often been overlooked in research on assisted and collaborative reproduction. Southern states may be assumed to be universally against reproductive technologies because such technologies

TABLE 6.1 Uniform Parentage Laws by State

	UPA 1973	UPA 2002	UPA 2017
AL	1984	2008	—
AK	—	—	—
AZ	—	—	—
AR	—	—	—
CA	1976	—	2018
CO	1977	—	—
CT	—	—	Introduced as of 2021
DE	—	2003	—
DC	—	—	—
FL	—	—	—
GA	—	—	—
HI	1976	—	—
ID	—	—	—
IL	1984	2015	—
IN	—	—	—
IA	—	—	—
KS	1985	—	—
KY	—	—	—
LA	—	—	—
ME	—	2015	Introduced as of 2021
MD	—	—	—
MA	—	—	—
MI	—	—	—
MN	1980	—	—
MS	—	—	—
MO	—	—	—
MT	1975	—	—
NE	—	—	—
NV	—	—	—
NH	—	—	—
NJ	1983	—	—
NM	—	2009	—
NY	—	—	—
NC	—	—	—
ND	1975	2005	—
OH	1983	—	—
OK	—	2006	—
OR	—	—	—
PA	—	—	Introduced as of 2021
RI	1983	—	2020
SC	—	—	—
SD	—	—	—
TN	—	—	—
TX	1989	2001	—

(*Continued*)

TABLE 6.1 (Continued)

	UPA 1973	UPA 2002	UPA 2017
UT	—	2005	—
VT	—	—	2018
VA	—	—	—
WA	1976	2002	2018
WV	—	—	—
WI	—	—	—
WY	—	2003	—
Total	14	11	4 (plus 3 introduced)

NOTES: "Introduced" means proposed UPA legislation was introduced for consideration but has not been passed or enacted into law.

are assumed to symbolically align with what Cahn and Carbone (2010, 3) describe as the "blue family paradigm," denoting more liberal or progressive ideologies about the changing American family. Yet southern states can offer additional insights into the cultural reception of the new reproductive technologies for two reasons. First, there is no monolithic southern culture that necessarily dictates how reproductive technologies are perceived in the South. Larry Griffin (2000) reminds us of the need to focus on southern cultures, despite the common representation in American public imagination of the South as a uniform region. For instance, one discovery I made in conducting research for this chapter is that legislators, physicians, and lobbyists in Louisiana (many of whom supported a socially conservative definition of "family") framed IVF and collaborative reproduction as both supporting and violating pro-life and pro-family ideologies. Legislators and bill proponents sympathetic to assisted and collaborative reproduction couched their arguments as supporting and protecting Louisiana families and having children who would not otherwise exist, while their opponents argued that these families were not being made according to what they called God's plan. Second, if we accept the premise that overall southern states are more conservative than other parts of the United States in terms of family politics (Cahn and Cambone 2010), then looking at those states more closely can give us a glimpse of the extent to which assisted and collaborative reproduction has become normalized in the United States. A state's taking action to regulate, as well as the type and content of those actions, can show just how much these technologies are perceived to undermine or affirm the traditional social and legal order.

Legal Parentage and Collaborative Reproduction

Questions about parentage in assisted and collaborative reproduction are integrally connected to other politically divisive issues, most notably abortion politics and the purported destruction of the traditional family. I described these above as the frames of politics of life and politics of family for IVF and AID, respectively. For AID, clarifying paternity and legally protecting the traditional family was the main social problem for courts and legislatures to address. During the first half of the twentieth century, AID was relatively unsettled as a legal issue. Before the 1960s, state-level activity occurred largely through a handful of court cases and often involved marital dissolution and subsequent disputes over men's rights and responsibilities in relation to a donor-conceived child. Most, but not all, of the court decisions upheld the notions that AID-conceived children were legitimate and that AID was not a form of adultery committed by the recipient wife. Although legislation on AID and paternity was proposed in a handful of states in the late 1940s (Schatkin 1954), the first statute on the subject (in Georgia) was not enacted until 1964 (Dolgin 1997). Oklahoma followed suit three years later, in 1967. Both statutes declared that AID-conceived children were legitimate children of their mother's husband, provided the husband had consented to the procedure.

In the next two decades, many states enacted similar laws. Although only a minority of states adopted the 1973 UPA, Gaia Bernstein (2002, 1090) notes that it provided both a catalyst and a "stabilizing force" for further state legislation on AID and paternity. The UPA included a section legalizing AID if the husband consented and absolving the sperm donor of any paternal rights or responsibilities (Bernstein 2002). This approach provided highly visible model legislation to expand legal paternity to encompass

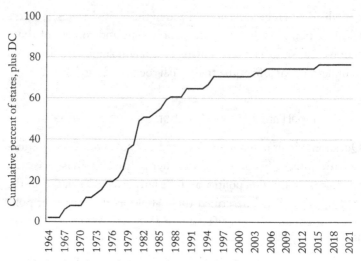

FIG. 6.1. Percentages of states with statutes on AID, 1964–2021

and normalize AID. As a result, there was a substantial increase in state-level action between 1970 and 1980 (Figure 6.1). By 1982, half of the states had enacted statutory laws on AID and paternity.

However, the legal impetus to address AID paternity largely plateaued in the 1990s and early 2000s. During this time there was also a general decline in the number of heterosexual couples using AID because of new technological developments that allowed many infertile men to use their own sperm (Spar 2006; Agigian 2004; Practice Committee of the American Society for Reproductive Medicine and Society for Assisted Reproductive Technology 2012). After these developments, perhaps state legislatures saw AID paternity as a less-urgent matter to attend to. Still, by 2015 more than three-fourths (76.5 percent) of all states plus the District of Columbia had enacted statutes on AID paternity (Nejaime 2017).[2]

What about the legal landscape for egg donation, embryo donation, and gestational surrogacy? IVF emerged on the heels of *Roe v. Wade* and made its U.S. debut early in a newly conservative political era that was ushered in by the administration of President Ronald Reagan and was strongly aligned with the fundamentalist Christian right (Midgley 1992; Stacey 1996). A new political narrative on 'family values' came to the forefront of political discussions and public imagination. Central to this narrative was the purported demise of the traditional family, allegedly evidenced by rising rates of abortion, single motherhood, divorce, and nonmarital births. Most important to the narrative, women and feminism were identified as the main culprits in the destruction of the American family (Stacey 1996). This social and political context was ripe for generating discussions about maternity and motherhood (Markens 2007; Rothman 1989) and pressure to regulate or restrict new reproductive technologies that challenged the traditional biological presumption of maternity.

Figure 6.2 shows state-level trends in the enactment of statutes governing egg donation, embryo donation, and gestational

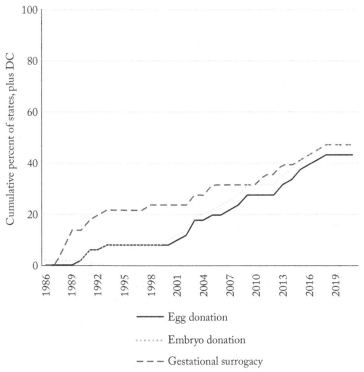

——— Egg donation

········ Embryo donation

– – – Gestational surrogacy

FIG. 6.2. Percentages of states with statutes on egg donation, embryo donation, and gestational surrogacy, 1986–2021

surrogacy. In 1986, Louisiana became the first state to enact a statute addressing parentage via embryo donation. Between 1986 and 2000, less than 10 percent of the states enacted any statute on egg or embryo donation maternity. This figured tripled by 2010. Some of this increase might be attributable to the 2000 UPA, which the ULC had updated to include, among other things, a formal section on various types of assisted and collaborative reproduction (ULC 2021b). The percentage of states adopting parentage statutes on egg and embryo donation and gestational surrogacy continued to slowly increase, but the overall trend has decidedly not matched the pace of adoption of AID paternity laws in the wake of the 1973 UPA. At the time of this writing, in early 2021, fewer than half of the states have statutory laws on egg donation or embryo donation maternity (43 percent and 47 percent, respectively: two states explicitly regulate embryo but not egg donation parentage). In an initial flurry of legislative activity in the late 1980s, likely in response to the Baby M[3] case, around one-fifth of the states passed laws on surrogacy. Most of these were restrictive, and many did not distinguish between traditional and gestational surrogacy. Several of these statutes (e.g., those in Washington and Utah) were later repealed and replaced by others that allowed gestational, but not traditional, surrogacy agreements. Trends generally converged for all three reproductive techniques during the early 2000s and 2010s. Currently, fewer than half of the states (47 percent) explicitly address gestational surrogacy in statutory law.

It is also important to note here the disjuncture between the laws 'on the books' and the "actual practice" of law (Hinson 2011, 36). Diane Hinson (2011) points out how gestational surrogacy practices vary for vacuum states—those with no case or statutory law to guide actions in this area. In these instances, much is left to the discretion of the courts. Some courts "routinely grant" prebirth orders to legally delineate parentage before a child's birth (e.g., before embryo transfer or just after confirmation of pregnancy); some courts have a history of allowing only post birth adoption proceedings to occur; and still others are "unpredictable" in terms of what if anything they would grant (Hinson and McBrien 2011, 35).

An additional significant point here is that while the data in Figure 6.2 provide an overview of state-level statutory trends, they gloss over the substantial variation in legal approaches by state. Some states have enacted comprehensive acts that cover a range of techniques in one fell swoop (e.g., Florida, in 1993). Others have taken a much more piecemeal approach, opting to address techniques one at a time or only some of the techniques. For example, Alabama enacted the 2000 version of the UPA in 2008 but left only a placeholder under Article 8 for gestational surrogacy. The article has a title but for now contains only the word "reserved." Statutes are not even reliably in similar chapters or titles of states' legal codes: some are listed under "vital statistics," others under "domestic relations," and still others under sections related to inheritance or public health and safety. Some states are on the forefront of regulating, taking general proactive measures; others are more reactive, perhaps creating law in response to localized disputes or dilemmas of particular constituents or events. Finally, an important difference appears in the specific content of the statutes—notably in who is treated as a natural parent and who would need to undergo adoption or another legal proceeding to be invested with parental rights; and whether the law sides with certain parties over others (e.g., privileging the rights of intended parents, genetic parents, or birth parents). It is no wonder that many scholars and journalists attempting to summarize and clarify U.S. law on assisted and collaborative reproduction use such language as "crazy quilt" and "patchwork." But other terms are also frequently used to describe these reproductive innovations and their relationship to law and society: frontier, pioneer, and brave new world. These terms hint that, for better or worse, the technologies are propelling us toward a new precipice of social and cultural change. How are legal actors making sense of this new "frontier" and its implications for maternity and the American family?

Of Embryos and Families: The Case of Louisiana

In 1986, Louisiana became the first state to enact legislation on IVF embryos and embryo donation parentage. To prevent excess

IVF-created embryos from languishing in frozen limbo or becoming scientific research material, the statute provided for embryo donation or adoption as a legally recognized form of parenthood. In 1987, the legislature also quickly enacted a statute making paid contracts for traditional surrogacy illegal in the state. This swift legislative action emerged in response to the ongoing national controversy over the Baby M case. It was authored by Representative Arthur Morrell (D), who later noted that his bill passed both the Louisiana House of Representatives and State Senate, "without a single dissenting vote" (as quoted in *Surrogacy Arrangements Act of 1987*, 101) and defined traditional surrogacy contracts as "absolutely null . . . void . . . [and] unenforceable as contrary to public policy" (Louisiana Revised Statute 1987). Not until 2000 did the Louisiana legislature address gestational surrogacy among biological family members. And it would take another sixteen years after that for the legislature to address gestational surrogacy among legal strangers. As of this writing, no legislation in Louisiana clarifies parentage via egg donation. Some readers might presume that egg donation arrangements would confer legal maternity on the gestational mother. In line with traditional understandings of embodied bio-legal maternity, Article 184 of the Louisiana Civil Code (2009) states that "maternity may be established by a preponderance of evidence[4] that the child was born of a particular woman, except otherwise provided by law." However, discussions emerging from the other statutes on collaborative reproduction hint that it might not be so simple—especially if a donor were to assert her own genetic maternity claims. This is all part of the complexities of maternity that I explore below.

It is worth mentioning briefly here that Louisiana is somewhat different from the rest of the country in terms of its legal tradition, which is rooted in civil law for private law, influenced by French, Spanish, and Roman tradition, but also includes public law and courts modeled on the U.S. common law system that was influenced by English tradition (Algero 2005; Hood 1958). Some major distinctions between civil law and common law include the extent to which they are codified, how general versus particular they are, and the weight they give to precedent (Algero 2005). Because I focus on the development, debate, and content of statutory law as opposed to case law in Louisiana, I argue that the distinct legal tradition of Louisiana does not necessarily make it unique in its approach to regulating IVF and collaborative reproduction.

PROTECTING THE "WEAKEST LINK": THE LOUISIANA HUMAN EMBRYO ACT (1986)

The 1986 Louisiana Human Embryo Act represented an early foray into state-level regulation of IVF in the United States. IVF was still in its nascent stages in the country, with the first U.S. IVF baby having been born only five years earlier, in Norfolk, Virginia. In Louisiana, the first 'certificate of need' for an IVF program was approved in 1983. The program was a joint effort between a community hospital and a private fertility clinic founded and directed by Dr. Richard Dickey (Dickey et al. 1984). Dickey was not new to infertility or women's health, having founded the New Orleans Fertility Institute in 1976 and before that having devoted his career to studying hormonal contraception. Of particular note, Dickey and Clyde Dorr (1969, 278) had studied contraceptives' side effects, confirming prior "impressions" of what women were anecdotally reporting. Dickey and Dorr cautioned about the "potential danger . . . of hormonal excess" to women's health, recommending lower dosages and more individualized patient prescriptions than were common then (281). At that time many women's concerns were ignored, downplayed, or not systematically attended to by either policy makers or medical and scientific professionals (Marks 1999). Dickey was an advocate of both IVF and women's reproductive health more broadly.[5]

Two years after Louisiana's first IVF program opened, John Krentel—then a law student at Loyola University—published a proposal to regulate IVF and assisted reproduction in Louisiana. Krentel bemoaned the lack of an "ethical framework . . . for responsible decision-making" in IVF (1985, 287). At the time, the Louisiana State Medical Society had not provided any explicit guidance on best practices in IVF. As I described in chapter 3, the

American Fertility Society (AFS) was only starting to fill this void in ethical guidance, releasing its first brief statement in 1984; its first in-depth report did not come until 1986 (AFS Committee on Ethics 1986). IVF and the pre-embryo had an uncertain ethical and legal status in the post-Roe era. If *Roe v. Wade* had made it clear that a fertilized ovum in utero was "akin to property of the pregnant woman"[6] (Krentel 1985, 284) how should the law consider an embryo outside of the maternal body? What rights or interests did it have?

IVF had already created substantial public and professional concern about its possibilities for interfering in human reproduction. There was also a major lapse in federal oversight for ethical guidance, creating a time of great uncertainty about the technology. IVF provided a political opportunity to address the disembodied embryo as a distinct entity. Political sociologists describe such opportunities as "sets of clues that encourage people to engage in contentious politics" (Tarrow 2011, 32). Pro-life activists strategically used this time of uncertainty about IVF to gain political traction across the country (Cromer 2019; Flavin 2008; Quigley and Andrews 1984). Thus it should not be surprising that the first version of the Louisiana bill was sponsored by Louisiana Right to Life (Dickey et al. 1995), a pro-life lobbying organization founded in 1970 whose mission is to "restore the right to life in Louisiana by opposing abortion, euthanasia, and other life destroying actions" (Louisiana Right to Life 2020).[7]

As a more general legal issue, legislative intent can be difficult to discern from the historical record. However, Krentel's intent was quite apparent. He argued that the in vitro fertilized embryo was the most vulnerable party in IVF because it was in legal and ethical limbo—was it property or a person? What considerations did physicians and courts owe to this "unique category of being," whose "radical link [to the] human form . . . cannot be denied" (1985, 287)? Krentel proposed establishing the IVF-created, disembodied embryo as a *juridical person*. While this legal status was usually reserved for nonhuman entities such as corporations or partnerships, using it in this instance would attribute personality[8] to the disembodied embryo, giving it a formal legal identity as well as certain protected rights and interests. Krentel further proposed that any excess embryos not implanted by the original IVF patients could not be destroyed or donated to science. They had to be stored indefinitely. Physicians would also be "directly responsible for the in vitro safekeeping of the fertilized ovum" and held to the "highest standard of care" (Krentel 1985, 288). Most of what Krentel originally proposed would become law under the Human Embryo Act (1986). Krentel (1999, 246) later observed: "this designation [as a juridical person] 'holds the line' against the erosion of respect for human life by safeguarding the weakest link in the human chain—the in vitro fertilized ovum."

Fearing that Krentel's original bill would not sufficiently protect physicians' ability to conduct IVF in Louisiana, Dr. Dickey became prominently involved in deliberations on the bill and redrafting efforts. This work included organizing a symposium that was jointly hosted by the Humana Women's Center at Humana Hospital and the Loyola Law School of New Orleans. The symposium focused on the morality of IVF, with a particular emphasis on the IVF-created embryo. Speaking about the "medical status of the embryo," Dickey (1986) expressed the need to respect the embryo but also the need to balance this respect with the practical needs of medicine and physicians' duty to their patients. He noted the strict protocol used at the Fertility Institute to transfer all IVF-created embryos back into the patient: "there is the basic recognition that all embryos are actual or potential human life. This position mandates the replacement of all embryos into the uterus, the only site in which they can develop to maturity" (330). One practical medical issue was that the IVF pregnancy rate relied on having enough good-quality embryos to transfer. Pregnancy rates increased with each additional embryo, although there were diminishing returns or sometimes negative effects when physicians transferred four or more embryos (Dickey 1986). Retrieving fewer eggs from patients was also risky. They might fail to be fertilized, requiring additional procedures. In the absence of viable long-term storage, there were only two outcomes for excess embryos:

transfer them all and risk a multiple pregnancy or have them go to waste. Considering these restricted options, Dickey argued that every IVF program should be prepared to have an "emergency embryo freezing procedure" in the future to "preserve the possibility of life for the embryo" (333).

Despite expressing concerns about the treatment and care of the IVF embryo, Dickey continually argued that IVF provided a "compassionate and ethical technological breakthrough" (1986, 336). In an impassioned statement with strong moral undertones, Dickey concluded: "[IVF] permits the human egg and sperm to complete the act for which they were intended, that is union and the reproduction of human life. If IVF were not done, eggs and sperm would be lost and the marital act would not only be ineffectual in achieving procreation but would be doubly frustrating to the married couple in that the marriage would be without hope of issue." IVF thus offered a way to preserve and protect early human life as well as the purpose of "the marital act."

The IVF symposium included two other participants to round out the discussion from religious and legal perspectives. Noting the need to balance "the life of the embryo against the chance to have a 'natural' child," the theologian Lisa Cahill (1986, 353) argued: "we are uncertain both how to define the value of [embryonic] life precisely and how to evaluate the seriousness of the problem of infertility in relation to other forms of human suffering. . . . I will venture to say that there is a moral obligation to minimize embryo loss, even if as a consequence the chance of pregnancy will not be optimal, and particularly if there is a diminishing rate of return with the escalation of numbers of transferrals."

Taking a different tack, Lori Andrews—a well-known feminist legal scholar whose analyses of reproductive technology frequently appeared in the pages of *Fertility and Sterility* and who had a seat on the AFS Committee on Ethics—argued that the parties whose rights were most at stake in the proposed Louisiana legislation were the patients, couples, and physicians, not the IVF-created embryo. She warned that physicians could be liable under a whole host of scenarios that might fall under the "highest standard of care" for the IVF-created embryo (1986a, 400). Furthermore, the proposed legislation created a forced choice: either a woman decided to have all the IVF-created embryos transferred into her uterus and risked having a multiple pregnancy and all the maternal and fetal complications that might bring, or she and her husband renounced their parental rights to their excess embryos. Andrews also argued that the statute violated couples' constitutional right to privacy in making procreative decisions because the state blocked them from having full dispositional control (to conceive, donate, or destroy) over their own reproductive materials. Although symbolic protection of the embryo could codify societal values about respect for the most vulnerable and for human life, this should not infringe on constitutionally protected rights. Andrews (1986a, 358) noted: "the law must be mindful of the tension between these two lines of precedents [protecting the embryo and protecting procreative autonomy]."

Both Andrew's invited presence at the symposium and her arguments about procreative autonomy provided notable challenges to focusing on embryonic life at the expense of the full-fledged people involved in IVF. However, her critique ultimately did little to slow the momentum of Krentel's work. In the end, both Dickey and Krentel gave formal support to a revision of the original proposal, which became Louisiana Senate Bill 701.[9] The bill formally granted juridical personality to IVF-created embryos, required that they had to be stored indefinitely or "adopted" by another married, heterosexual couple, and vested the overseeing physician with "temporary guardianship" of the disembodied embryos should "adoptive" parents need to be found (Senate Bill [SB] 701 1986a). In any disputes concerning the embryo (e.g., if the couple divorced before implantation), courts should decide based on the "best interests of the in vitro fertilized ovum" (SB 701 1986a). The bill passed the state senate thirty-seven to zero and passed the house eighty-three to thirteen. It was officially enacted as the Human Embryo Act (1986).

The act explicitly emerged from a politics of life framing of IVF. As evidenced by the topic of the symposium, as well as the name and content of the act, the purpose of the act seemingly had everything to do with embryos and little to do with parentage or maternity. Yet the act had substantial implications for thinking about maternity in the Louisiana context. Accounting for either reimplantation into the original patient or adoption by another couple as possible outcomes, the act both created a newly defined path for family building through embryo adoption and loosened the stronghold of the biological presumption of maternity in establishing legal maternity. However, I suggest that this new mode of family building was really a by-product of centering embryo personhood, rather than evidence that assisted reproduction was becoming more normalized in Louisiana at the time. Allowing for embryos to be adopted aligned with pro-life rhetoric that adoption was morally superior to abortion. In the context of IVF, embryo adoption was the moral solution compared to destroying embryos or donating them for scientific research.

Intriguingly, another by-product of the act was that it made it possible to argue that giving birth was not a foolproof way to establish maternity. Married couples who agreed to adoptive implantation would still need to undergo adoption proceedings after the birth occurred. The IVF-created embryo that had been created by not yet implanted was a liminal but also curiously autonomous entity. The progenitors of the conjugal embryo were prioritized in making parental claims to the embryo, but their parentage was not inevitable. According to the act, if the IVF patient and her husband "expressed their [parental] identity," those rights "[would] be preserved" (Human Embryo Act 1986). However, failure to "express" a parental identity meant that the overseeing physician became the "temporary guardian" of the embryo until "adoptive implantation can occur." But "adoptive implantation" also required more than a gestational relationship to establish maternity. Simply putting an embryo into another woman's body did not make her the legal mother of the subsequent child. Even as the act was clearly trying to reinforce a variant of the repronormative family by only allowing married heterosexual couples to adopt embryos, it represented a clear deviation from the traditional definition of maternity: giving birth was no longer sufficient proof in all scenarios. If simply disembodying an embryo for IVF created some degree of maternity uncertainty, what would happen when third parties were intentionally used to assist with reproduction?

AN ACT OF FAMILY LOVE

In 2000, Representative Sydnie Mae Durand (D) introduced Louisiana House Bill 181. This bill proposed to amend Louisiana's vital statistics laws, allowing genetic parents to be listed on the birth certificate if they used a blood relative for a gestational surrogate. The bill explicitly defined "biological parents" of the child as arising from the following conditions: "A husband and wife, joined by legal marriage recognized as valid in this state, who provide sperm and egg for in vitro fertilization, performed by a licensed physician, where the resulting fetus is carried and delivered by a surrogate birth parent who is a blood relative of either the husband or wife" (House Bill [HB] 181 2000a). When introducing or defending the bill on the House Floor, Durand repeatedly noted: "This bill probably represents what I think exemplifies the real meaning of family love" (HB 181 2000b). This framing firmly placed intrafamilial surrogacy in the realm of family and altruism and distanced it from the contentious issues associated with commercial surrogacy that many reproductive scholars have identified (Berend 2016; Jacobson 2016; Markens 2007). Durand went on to describe the main impetus for the bill, further drawing on the moral frame of the "plight of infertile couples" that the sociologist Susan Markens (2007, 81) identified in her work on surrogacy. A young couple who had been married for just a few years had no hope of having children on their own because the wife "was born without a uterus." The couple saw a fertility specialist and used IVF to create embryos from their own gametes, but they would also need a gestational surrogate. They identified the husband's sister as a candidate, who, Durand noted, also happened to be "[the wife's] best friend since grade school." According to Durand, everything was going according to plan until the couple was about to leave the hospital with their new baby: "all hell broke loose. . . . The medical people at the hospital . . . told [the family] that the birth certificate could have only the surrogate mother." The couple tried to explain that they were the biological [genetic] parents, but to no avail, and it became "necessary for them to adopt their own child" (HB 181 2000b).

Durand's bill sought to correct what she framed as a procedural mistake: the hospital's recognizing as the natural mother the gestational surrogate, instead of the genetic mother. The fact that this bill sought to amend only the vital statistics law reinforced the view that this was a mistaken understanding of maternity. The traditional legal presumption of maternity in this case was simply in error: it was out of sync with the 'natural' facts. The bill overtly relied on a genetic definition of parentage. In several instances, Durand distinguished between traditional and gestational surrogacy, noting that the traditional surrogate was truly a mother (because her egg was used) but clarifying that this was not the type of surrogacy she was aiming to regulate with her bill. Discussing the bill on the floor of the Louisiana House, Durand underscored this point: "I didn't say surrogate mother, and I want to make sure you understand the difference. The difference is that a surrogate mother is the person who donates the egg [referring to traditional surrogacy], while a gestational carrier is a woman who carries another woman's embryo for nine months. So, in other words, [the gestational carrier] acts as the incubator" (HB 181 2000b). The reference to the gestational carrier as an "incubator" is a specific description of surrogacy that feminist scholars have heavily criticized, arguing that it downplays the significant contribution of the gestational role as well as demoting pregnant women from full human beings to wombs and gestators (Lublin 1998; Rothman 1989; Thompson 2002). But this was not a misstep. By using the term "incubator," Durand strategically sought to elevate one woman's maternal status above another's.

Durand also later corrected a questioning colleague who referred to a "surrogate mother" instead of a "gestational carrier." She reminded her colleague that the egg and sperm did not come from anonymous gamete donors but from a married couple, "the husband and wife" who had created the conjugal embryo (HB 181 200b):

REP. DOWNER: Under current law, the only individual who can be on the birth certificate . . . is the surrogate mother?

REP. DURAND: Yes, who was not a surrogate *mother* [in this case], she was a carrier. . . .

REP. DOWNER: The surrogate mother is different. . . . I appreciate [that there is a difference]. In definition, the surrogate mother is an individual who is fertilized by the natural father.

REP. DURAND: Right.

REP. DOWNER: Using her own egg?

REP. DURAND: Right.

REP. DOWNER: This [bill] provides [for cases] where we have a donor who is the natural parent of the egg, and the donor of the sperm.

REP. DURAND: The husband and wife.

House Bill 181 could correct the error of bestowing legal maternity on the surrogate, allowing the 'natural' (i.e., genetic, married) parents instead to be listed on the birth certificate. It also did not require legal recognition of the gestational carrier on any paperwork. DNA testing was required after the baby was born to confirm that it was in fact the genetic child of the married couple and not the surrogate. The bill was ultimately enacted into law, passing both the House (ninety-five to five votes) and the Senate (a hundred to zero) with very little controversy or discussion. This indicated a perhaps rare political and moral consensus on intrafamilial gestational surrogacy in the Louisiana legislature.

How should we interpret the statute? From one perspective, we could read its enactment as a win for genetic maternity. Referring to the genetic mother as the real mother, citing DNA as scientific proof of maternity, and referring to the gestational surrogate as an "incubator" all elevate genetics above gestation. But the situation is also more complicated because it is not just about genetics versus gestation. The statute explicitly defines biological parenthood as arising from heterosexual marriage. The conjugal embryo is crucial to sorting out parentage claims. Additionally, the statute applies only when the gestational carrier is a blood relative of the husband or wife. Rep. Durand repeatedly described intra-familial gestational surrogacy as an "act of real family love." This framed such surrogacy both as an altruistic act, which other researchers have noted regarding surrogacy in general (Ragone 1999; Jacobson 2016), and one that was largely regulated within the quasi-private realm of the family. Familial relationships are presumed to be based on personal and affective ties and moral obligations, juxtaposed with commercialization and contracts, and the latter are often framed as antithetical to, and potentially contaminating of, the former (Zelizer 2000). As Representative Hebert summed up in supporting the bill, "because of that family bond and the love in that family, his sister agreed to be implanted . . . and to carry that baby and to have that baby for her brother and his wife . . . [A]ll Miss Sydnie Mae [Rep. Durand] is trying to do with her bill is help this couple out" (HB 181 2000b). This view, that intra-familial gestational surrogacy was first and foremost about "family love," seemed to justify both the morality of this type of collaborative reproduction and the minimal state intervention in sorting out parentage—requiring only an amendment to vital statistics law to correct the 'facts' of the situation.

The philosopher Charis Thompson's (2005, 145) work on "disambiguat[ing]" kinship also points to the role of the incest taboo in regulating parentage when family members serve as donors or surrogates. When the husband's sister serves as a gestational surrogate (as in the case that prompted Durand's bill), recognizing her maternity would place her in a seemingly incestuous relationship with her brother. Thus, downplaying any semblance of incest is also at stake. While incest may act as an implicit taboo, regulating the family sphere, it also operates formally in laws. Louisiana explicitly defines marital or sexual relations between siblings as a "crime against nature" (Louisiana Revised Statute 2018). Although IVF is medicalized and asexual, placing the surrogate sister on the birth certificate with the sperm provider brother might suggest a sexual relationship between siblings. Declaring the married genetic parents as the 'real' parents allows the sibling relationship to resume its moral, nonsexual form.

What about the status of the disembodied IVF embryo, which was so central to the 1986 Human Embryo Act? In contrast to this earlier act, the 2000 statute did not undermine the intended parents' claims by disembodying the embryo. The intended parents did not lose their automatic and naturally assumed parental rights by putting their conjugal embryo into the surrogate sister's body—unlike the IVF patients whose disembodied conjugal embryo was put under physician guardianship and considered eligible for adoption if they did not express parental interests in it. The tenacity of the intended parents' rightful claim to parentage in Durand's bill was further underscored by the explicit lack of acknowledgment of the birth maternity of the gestational surrogate sister. According to the bill, the sister did not even need to appear on the child's birth certificate. Such an approach reinforced the view that maternity and parentage 'naturally' flowed from genetics and the conjugal embryo. But what if the surrogate was not a blood relative of one of the intended parents? What if she was a legal stranger to them? Who were the natural parents then? The Louisiana legislature would wait at least another decade to take up this issue.

ADOPTING THEIR OWN CHILD

It was not until 2016 that the Louisiana legislature enacted a statute addressing nonfamilial gestational surrogacy. By the mid-2010s IVF and its variants (egg donation, embryo donation, and gestational surrogacy) were substantially more normalized in the United States compared to previous decades. As the sociologist and anthropologist Sarah Franklin (2013, 1) argued, by then IVF had become "routine and familiar. . . . [A] normal fact of life." Yet it was not just the passage of time that had helped create a political atmosphere accepting of collaborative reproduction. In Louisiana, a nonfamilial gestational surrogacy bill had been introduced twice before (in 2013 and 2014) and had been passed by the state's House and Senate. Although the bill had bipartisan support and was cosponsored by Democrat and Republican legislators, pro-life

Governor Bobby Jindal (R) vetoed it both times, citing "serious concern from various groups across the state" (Jindal 2013).[10] In 2015, Louisiana citizens elected a new, Democratic governor, John Bel Edwards. Like many southern Democrats, Edwards was pro-life and generally socially conservative. Yet, Edwards also sought to clearly distinguish himself from his predecessor, overturning many of Jindal's policy decisions (e.g., Edwards opted to expand eligibility for Medicaid under the Affordable Care Act). The change in administration provided a political opportunity: House Bill 1102, which regulated nonfamilial gestational carrier contracts, was signed into law in 2016.

Although the new law was characterized as a "modest" and "conservative" step (House Bill [HB] 1102 2016b) relative to laws in other states, it officially legalized nonfamilial gestational surrogacy agreements. It also provided a specific sequence of events for use in clarifying parentage. Prior to any embryo transfer procedures, the intended parents, the gestational surrogate, and her husband (if she was married) would need to initiate proceedings for a court-approved contract. The contract had specific conditions (HB 1102 2016a): all parties had to have lived in Louisiana for at least 180 days, the intended parents had to be married to each other[11] and use their own gametes, and a state-licensed physician certified in reproductive medicine had to sign an affidavit that surrogacy was medically necessary for the intended mother to have a child. After background checks showed that none of the parties had a criminal record, a court would order a hearing at which it would declare that the intended parents were, in fact, the legal parents of any resulting child. Then, after the embryo transfer and a successful pregnancy, the intended parents had to obtain a post-birth order,[12] for which they had to present a certified copy of the child's original birth certificate (which listed the gestational surrogate as the mother). This order would prompt the state to issue a new birth certificate listing the intended parents. However, the original birth certificate would still exist as a legal document, "sealed and subject to release or inspection" if there was any "good cause" to require it (Louisiana Revised Statute 2016). This process is analogous to the closed system of contemporary U.S. adoption law, according to which original birth certificates and other records pertaining to adoption are sealed and a second birth certificate issued, using the names of the adoptive parents instead of those of the birth parents (Cahn 2009 and 2013). The similarity to adoption was not a coincidence. Official revision comments in the history and commentary of the statute describe the process required for nonfamilial gestational surrogacy as "roughly analogous to prevailing adoption procedures. Just as adoption contemplates the transfer of parentage [from birth to adoptive parents] . . . a gestational carrier contract involves the transfer from the gestational mother to the intended parents" (Louisiana Official Revision Comments 2017).

Sponsors and supporters of the bill raised the issue of needing to protect Louisiana families using gestational surrogacy. Notably, not all families could qualify for such protection. Clearly invoking the repronormative family, the bill applied only to married heterosexual couples using their own gametes. These restrictions prompted opposition from Equality Louisiana and Louisiana Trans Advocates. Supporters framed the bill as a way to provide much-needed regulation for otherwise traditional families who simply had to have extra help to have a biological child. The supporters also aimed to move the discussion away from the ethics of IVF and the politics of life framing that had been so central to the 1986 Human Embryo Act.

Presenting the bill in the House Committee on Civil Law and Procedure, Representative Stuart Bishop (R) said: "This bill is not creating a law. [IVF is] already legal. . . . [The bill is] creating a contract that protects four people: the intended parents, the gestational carrier, and the child" (HB 1102 2016c). Later on in the same committee hearing, Katherine Smith, a Louisiana state senator's wife and infertility patient, provided personal testimony in support of the bill, focusing the conversation on the moral acts involved in family building and wanting to have a biological child: "[This bill] protects not only couples who find themselves in the predicament that Gary and I found ourselves in: wanting a family and willing to go to extraordinary lengths to have biological children. But it will also protect those gestational carriers who choose to help those couples" (HB 1102 2016d).

Bill supporters argued that intended parents using gestational surrogacy in Louisiana were at risk of not being recognized as legal parents because they had to resort to "adopting their own child" in the absence of clear statutes regulating non-familial gestational surrogacy. As Representative Lopinto (R) underscored in presenting the bill before the House Committee on Civil Law and Procedure: "The premise behind this bill is very simple. Should a mother and father, using their own DNA, have to adopt their own child? . . . This [bill lays out] a contract [to address this]. . . . The only procedure in Louisiana [before the proposed court-approved contract and post-birth order] is they had to adopt their own child [after birth]. If that surrogate mother . . . decides they're going to change their mind and they're not going to give that child up for adoption, there's nothing that those parents can do. . . . They're—they're stuck" (HB 1102 2016e).

Supporters repeatedly used the phrase "adopting their own child" to emphasize the irony of biological parents' not having immediate rights to their "own" children. In the Western cultural context, it is indeed unnatural to have to adopt your own child—an inherent violation of the natural, moral order of the family (Dolgin 1997; Schneider 1984). Adoption is what you do to acquire legal parentage of other people's children, not your own.[13] This framing of the bill, similar to that of the 2000 statute, presented the problem as one of disjuncture between the legal and natural facts of parentage. For instance, Smith, reading a prepared statement in multiple committee hearings, described how she and her husband Gary (a Louisiana state senator and original sponsor of the 2013 bill) had decided to use gestational surrogacy after receiving the "mind blowing" and "heart wrenching" news that she had only one fallopian tube and essentially "half of a uterus" (HB 1102 2016d and 2016i). Referring to the disjuncture between legal and natural parentage, Smith further noted that she and her husband had opted to go out of state to have their two children because "the law in Louisiana says that the woman who delivers the child is considered the mother regardless of whether the DNA of that child proves otherwise."

In additional personal testimony in support of the bill, Loren McIntyre—an infertility patient speaking about her own experiences with needing gestational surrogacy—said she believed that the current legal status of gestational surrogacy in Louisiana undermined both her claims to her conjugal genetic child and the integrity of her family unit. Showing a picture of her child to the committee members, she stated: "this is 100% genetically our child: the embryo was made from my egg and my husband's sperm. . . . [W]e knew [in Louisiana] that I was going to have to legally adopt my child and at the time we were told that my husband would be placed on the birth certificate as the biological father. [Later] . . . the hospital told us that they were not willing to put my husband on the birth certificate because [the gestational carrier] was a married woman" (HB 1102 2016f).

McIntyre and her husband found another hospital for the delivery—one that would put her husband's name on the birth certificate—but she still felt marginalized during the experience, with her own maternity unrecognized: "when it came time to put a hospital bracelet on both the baby and my husband, [it] beared [*sic*] the last name of our gestational carrier. I was not allowed to have a hospital bracelet for my own genetic child. . . . [Six months later] we're currently in the process of waiting to formally adopt him. . . . As my son's birth certificate currently reads, it lists our gestational carrier as the mother and my husband as the father" (HB 1102 2016f). McIntyre's testimony spoke to how the legal situation in Louisiana disrupted multiple families by refusing to recognize genetics as the basis of parentage. The hospital bracelet and the birth certificate both operated here as symbols of family constellations. Because McIntyre had not been allowed to have a hospital bracelet, she viewed herself as relationally disconnected from her genetic child: her maternity was made invisible in the hospital. Additionally, linking the gestational carrier (a married woman) and the genetic father (the husband of McIntyre, the genetic mother) in parentage through their shared hospital bracelets and the birth certificate further violated the boundaries not just of the genetic family of the intended parents, but also of the gestational surrogate's conjugal family.

Overall, proponents of the bill argued in favor of recognizing the genetic, conjugal family as the clear, natural family unit, saying that the law needed to be corrected to reflect and protect this family constellation. However, opponents strongly criticized this position for relying too narrowly on genetic maternity and ignoring family bonds and family creation more holistically. While the list of opponents included representatives seeking family equality for LGBT families so they could also use gestational surrogacy (and donor gametes), the most vocal opponents came from more conservative organizations that framed surrogacy as an unnatural practice that sought to disrupt the traditional family.

Representing the Louisiana Family Forum, whose tagline is "your voice for traditional families," (Louisiana Family Forum 2022), the organization's president, Gene Mills, argued that surrogacy contracts violated the "integrity of the family" and undermined the biological presumption of maternity. Allowing surrogacy contracts would create a slippery slope leading toward "relegating motherhood to a disposable status": "[In surrogacy a] child is born outside of a natural arrangement and birth mothers who consent . . . to bear a child and then forfeit the child before the child is even conceived. . . . In Louisiana, the long-standing assumption has always been . . . the woman who bears and delivers the child is indeed the mother of that child. . . . You're going to take away that presumption of every birth . . . and now that will be a legal question" (HB 1102 2016g). Mills also argued that simply contributing an egg did not (and should not) make women into mothers at the expense of birth mothers' parental rights: "The woman who contributes the egg by contract becomes the mother of the child. The birth mother, before any action is taken, relinquishes her rights of [sic] the child long before the child is actually artificially conceived."

Similarly, Alana Newman—director of the Coalition against Reproductive Trafficking, an organization opposed to all forms of collaborative reproduction—argued that gestational surrogacy contracts used "legal force to break natural bonds" between mothers and children (HB 1102 2016j). Surrogacy, according to Newman, was tantamount to "chopping up mothers into modular, separable pieces." Newman argued that if AID had made "disposable" fathers, surrogacy created "disposable motherhood," and it would not be long before the fertility industry would create its "true cash cow . . . [the] completely motherless child" (HB 1102 2016j). Newman's opposition to surrogacy, like that of several bill opponents, was not only opposition to fragmented motherhood and destruction of the relationship between the birth mother and child, but also opposition to what she viewed as the ultimate commodification of reproduction and family. The repronormative family was a quickly eroding barrier to cultural and social change, with integrated biosocial maternity as one of the last preserves.

Drawing comparisons to other disrupted family bonds, opponents of the bill argued that adoption was a moral family-building practice because it "redeem[ed] an imperfect situation" (HB 1102 2016g). However, collaborative reproduction intentionally disrupted the bond between the birth mother and child, thus inherently undermining the morality of families created in such a way. As Newman noted before the Committee on Judiciary B: "Children are good, families are good, but not all forms of conception are" (HB 1102 2016j). Similarly, Mills, in his testimony before Civil Law and Procedure, stated: "I caution you that while every child is made in the image and likeness of God, not every child is conceived according to the design or the plan of God. Commercial contracts for third party pregnancy have a potential to violate God's plan for procreation" (HB 1102 2016g). Finally, Charlotte Bergeron, President of Baton Rouge Right to Life, argued that there were "deep-rooted conflicts that are impossible to fix when we attempt to create human life through contracts between strangers" (HB 1102 2016k). Despite vocal and consistent opposition from organizations and individuals who were pro-life or supported so-called family values, the bill passed both the House (in a vote of eighty-five to fourteen) and the Senate (thirty to six) and was signed into law by Governor Edwards in 2016.

Maternity and Families in (Conflicting) Transition?

The trajectory of and debates surrounding these three Louisiana statutes represent both continuity and contradiction in how different actors and stakeholders were making sense of collaborative reproduction, family, and maternity. Some clear continuities throughout the period include the focus on the repronormative family as the type of family the state should support and legitimate and the emphasis on the conjugal embryo. This emphasis effectively restricted legally protected use of IVF and collaborative reproduction to married heterosexual couples using their own gametes to have a family and reinforced the married heterosexual prerogative in family building. Additionally, throughout the various debates, both the politics of life and the politics of family frames emerge, although sometimes one becomes more salient and emphasized than the other in how stakeholders framed the issues at hand. In the 1985–1986 debates and the resulting statute, the politics of life frame was front and center as the major justification for the bill. However, in the debates over the 2000 statute, this frame faded into the background. Only one legislator briefly brought up the status of the embryo during the House floor debate on the bill, but this did not prompt any further discussion. Instead, the primary focus was on the family and sorting out the natural and legal parentage in cases when a sister served as a surrogate for a married, heterosexual couple.

The 2016 statute saw a reemergence of both frames, combined with more of an explicit reckoning of how they did or did not fit together in the larger context of discourse on family values. Those who supported the bill sought to frame nonfamilial gestational surrogacy agreements as pro-family, arguing that the bill offered a way to help support and protect otherwise traditional Louisiana families. In the face of vocal opposition from those focusing on a politics of life frame, supporters emphasized the morality of assisted and collaborative reproduction in family building. Expressing frustration with bill opponents and sharing his own family's experience with infertility and assisted reproduction, Representative Tanner

Magee (R) summed up what he viewed as conflicting ideas of being pro-family and pro-life in the debate over the bill: "I can't help but think that if the people on the opposition side of the table had their way, that my children wouldn't be here today. . . . [W]hat's 'right to life'? . . . I have life because of [IVF]. . . . [S]o it's hard for me to sit here and say that I'm taking the 'right to life' position in opposing this bill because . . . [then] I wouldn't have [my] children" (HB 1102 2016h).

During the thirty-year period of debates on the different statutes, there were also contradictions in how different actors and stakeholders were making sense of collaborative reproduction, family, and maternity. Discussions about and the content of each of the statutes show different logics operating in terms of what legal actors were trying to accomplish (e.g., protecting embryos, establishing new forms of legal parentage, and protecting or restricting IVF). These different logics created some conflicting ideas about what exactly constituted maternity. Similar to the issues I described in chapter 4, neither genetics nor gestation was sufficient on its own to definitively establish maternity. However, Louisiana laws created even further contingencies in cases of post-IVF maternities. Both genetics and gestation emerged as major components, but their significance was situated in the larger web of relationships that had to be considered: intrafamilial versus non-familial ones, as well as relationships to the disembodied and variously reembodied embryo.

As a "ruby red" state in the South (Bridges 2020), Louisiana is a case that provides insights into legislative grappling with IVF, collaborative reproduction, and the family. Lawmakers aimed to retain the centrality of the traditional family as a moral and legal unit while expanding the accepted paths to family building. In other words, they were increasingly embracing postmodern family building, but not postmodern family forms. As Carolyn Michelle (2006) and Maureen Baker (2005) both show in their work on IVF, these newer reproductive technologies have the socially disruptive potential to expand access to family building and new family forms, but they can also be circumscribed to support the status quo. In the case of Louisiana, these technologies were largely framed and deployed in service of reproducing the traditional family, but with a little bit of help from physicians and collaborative parties. Questions about maternity and maternity uncertainty were woven throughout debates on the various bills but not always central, in large part because lawmakers were not thinking just about maternity as a specific relationship—they were thinking about the family as a social whole, not a collection of autonomous individuals with different interests and relationships to one another (Dolgin 1997). In this context, lawmakers could both adopt and resist new forms of maternity along the way, based on its seeming congruence with their concept of family. Legislative activities, such as the ones I described above, do not just require working through the technical details and anticipating all the hypothetical scenarios that the new reproductive technologies might create. Rather, these efforts are much more fundamentally about whether and how collaborative reproduction is understood as compatible (or not) with the prevailing legal and social order.

7

Concluding Thoughts

Maternity Somewhere in Between

I began this book with the notion that maternity in the post-IVF era is rife with uncertainty. This uncertainty is a direct product of the way that IVF facilitates the movement of reproductive cells outside of and between bodies. While some of this cellular mobility also happens for sperm and thus affects paternity, the implications for maternity are quite distinct. The primary users of sperm donation as a solution for infertility are no longer married heterosexual couples but lesbian couples and single women seeking parenthood without a male partner (Agigian 2004; Spar 2006). The introduction and uptake of ICSI in the late 1980s and 1990s and various ways to extract sperm from infertile men has pushed treatment options for male infertility toward a reconsolidation of biological and social paternity (Kamischke and Nieschlag 1999; Practice Committee of the American Society for Reproductive Medicine and Society for Assisted Reproductive Technology 2012). In contrast, IVF created a paradigm shift most specifically for the treatment of women's infertility, moving fertilization outside of women's bodies. Later technological developments built on the disembodied reproductive framework of IVF, replacing other parts of the reproductive process with donor eggs, donor embryos, and gestational surrogacy. As a result, disembodied fertilization through IVF made it possible to fragment the different biological components of maternity into more pieces than was the case with AID and paternity (Guttmacher, Haman, and MacLeod 1950). In the post-IVF era, maternity as a legal and cultural construct is in flux. Maternity that is unmoored wholly or partially from its biological base becomes uncertain and contingent. These characteristics also help expose maternity as something that results from social and legal decision making.

Furthermore, this contingent and uncertain maternity is not unique but part of the broader landscape of postmodern families and family building. Hegemonic ideologies of family are being slowly dismantled with the increased visibility of diverse family forms and ways of building families (Stacey 1996). And to borrow from Andrew Cherlin's (2004) work on the American family, uncertainty is characteristic of a sort of deinstitutionalization of maternity: changing social norms about what does and should constitute maternity if we can no longer take for granted and solely rely on biological presumption. Of course, this does not apply to all reproductive scenarios. There are many situations in which the biological presumption works smoothly and appropriately to facilitate legal and social recognition of a mother-child relationship. At the same time, IVF and collaborative reproductive challenge the existing institution of motherhood. This challenge creates space for recognizing a wider array of mother-child relationships, but these various relationships also lack consistent social and legal protection. In this way post-IVF forms of maternity are an "incomplete institution" (Cherlin 1978).

When Cherlin proposed the concept of an "incomplete institution," he suggested that we might look particularly at custom, language, and law as evidence of tension and conflict about emerging social forms and scenarios. In assisted and collaborative reproduction, the legal and social presumption of biology is disrupted. This "habitualized" or "routiniz[ed]" action of legal tradition no longer works for all reproductive scenarios—particularly for those involving IVF and collaborative reproduction (Cherlin

1978, 636). The law has not responded uniformly or universally to the challenges posed by collaborative reproduction, creating an uneven landscape across the states (and even within some states) in terms of which types of maternities are clarified and protected. Thus, the law currently offers "incomplete institutional support" (Cherlin 1978, 645) for such collaborative family building. Incomplete institutions also suffer from "linguistic inadequacies . . . the absence of widely accepted definitions for . . . roles and relationships" (644). These inadequacies permeate fragmented maternity in terms of naming the different parties involved in collaborative reproduction: intended mother, gestational mother, surrogate mother, genetic mother, birth mother, social mother, and legal mother. The term "mother" here is not a self-contained status but a set of conditional statements. It is contingent and dependent on context. Maternity through collaborative reproduction becomes a situational accomplishment (West and Zimmerman 1987; West and Fenstermaker 1993), emerging through social situations— especially interactions with legal and medical institutions—as opposed to being inherent in the maternal-child dyad. The biological presumption of maternity and the repronormative family continue to act as cultural resources used to interpret new situations of maternity uncertainty. But as I have showed in the preceding chapters, they do not always provide clear or ethical ways to define maternity for a given child.

The sociologist Patricia Yancey Martin (2004, 1257) reminds us that social institutions are "inconsistent, contradictory, and rife with conflict." Although endurance over time is one of their main features, these institutions are also constantly changing. In a similar vein, Judith Stacey (1996, 7) described postmodern families as a "pastiche of old and new." In her work on gay and lesbian kinship, Kath Weston (1991) articulated two different types of kinship: biological and chosen families. Biologically fragmented maternity lies somewhere in between these kinship systems. It is familiar but also "unsettle[ing]" to the institutions of motherhood and family (P. Martin 2004, 1257). Weston (1991, 5) further noted:

"the material and emotional consequences that hinge upon which interpretation of kinship [choice or biology] prevails are truly far-reaching." Definitions of family matter. They influence real people's lives.

What, then, are the options for defining maternity moving forward? One option is to resist change and remain tied to the old order of maternity, using the biological presumption as the default. This is fraught with problems, though: Does the biological presumption refer specifically to pregnancy and birth? Or does it mean fully integrated genetic and gestational maternity? A second option is to relax the strict requirements of the biological presumption, but only if the other parts of the repronormative family constellation are there to create the whole assemblage. If we refuse to adopt a more comprehensive and expansive framework, maternity remains contingent—contradictory, conflicting, and uncertain because its silent (sometimes not so silent) referent remains fully integrated biosocial maternity. Operating under this old order but extending the framework just a bit (e.g., by recognizing parentage rights only for heterosexual families using conjugal embryos) leaves other family iterations without consistent legal protections in the post-IVF era. A third option is to embrace these newer possibilities for maternal-child relationships but also recognize the need to look to the state for external legitimation and support in granting and shoring up rights and responsibilities and protecting family integrity. Families need affective commitments and support from their members in daily living, as well as stability and support from other social institutions.

As I finished writing this book, two legal cases made headlines. A "throuple"[1] in California succeeded in having three fathers listed on the birth certificates of their two children, born with the use of donor embryos and gestational surrogacy. This was a legal act that had no precedent in the state, so the judge hearing the case initially told the fathers that they would need to "have a law passed or appeal" (quoted in Feldman 2020). After hearing the "tearful testimonies" from each of the men about their family-building journey and parental desires, the judge found a way to "use existing laws to give us the first birth certificate of its kind anywhere." In a second, highly publicized case, also in California, the actress Sofia Vergara and her former fiancé, Nick Loeb, battled for control of embryos they had frozen from IVF procedures while they were still together. Legal actions began in 2016, with Vergara suing Loeb so that Loeb could not use the frozen embryos to have a child via gestational surrogacy. The case proceeded largely in terms of breach of contract because the two had originally signed a contract that any use of the embryos required written consent from both parties (City News Service 2021). In response to Vergara's suit, Loeb filed suit in Louisiana—hoping to use the provisions of the 1986 Human Embryo Act to limit Vergara's control over the embryos (by having them redefined as 'juridical persons'). The Los Angeles Superior Court decided Vergara's suit in her favor, and Loeb's Louisiana suit was dismissed.

Both of these two cases were considered newsworthy in part because they had sensational elements—a throuple of men having children together or a celebrity embattled with her ex. But these cases also give the public a glimpse into the legal complexities of families that do not fit neatly into repronormative family ideology and show how embryos become contentious entities, both symbolically and practically. The first case gives some cause for optimism by showing the creative possibilities of the law to protect a variety of family forms and family-building routes. However, such an outcome is highly dependent on finding a sympathetic judge and having legal options and the resources to take advantage of those options. The law can be used creatively, but relying on individualized, case-by-case strategies and appeals does not equitably protect vulnerable and marginalized people and family building in the way that more comprehensive regulation could. Feminist scholars have articulated the limits and pitfalls of collaborating with the state to advance social justice and social change (Luna and Luker 2013; Kim 2020). But they have also critiqued the issues with leaving reproductive rights in the realm of privacy and individual choice (Price 2010; Luna and Luker 2011)—a discursive and legal space that typically only furthers stratified reproduction (Colen

1995). Using the state as a tool to protect families is rife with concern, but leaving families without institutional support is not an option.

The second case speaks directly to control of the disposition of IVF-created embryos in case of relationship dissolution as well as the general need to carefully consider disembodied embryos in larger conversations about reproductive rights and reproductive justice. Feminist and family scholars have to take seriously discussions about the moral and legal status of the disembodied, IVF-created embryo. In this vein, the anthropologist Risa Cromer (2019) describes the rise of and ensuing shift in the personhood movement over the twentieth century, from little public perception of personhood before birth to substantial political action within the pro-life movement to recognize fetuses, and later embryos, as natural persons. Yet while Cromer notes that prior feminist scholarship (e.g., Petchesky 1987) focused on the "discursive untethering of embryos from maternal bodies" (Cromer 2019, 26) to make embryos appear as "autonomous entities," the IVF-created embryo is both discursively and physically untethered. Disembodied moments in assisted and collaborative reproduction give the embryo a strange, liminal status in which it is both autonomous from, but utterly dependent on, a maternal body for its development. How should the embryo be legally classified while disembodied? Should we grant intended parents property rights to embryos? Should we grant parentage rights for embryos? The answers to these questions might seem to solve the immediate problems for maternity and parentage disputes. But they also have much broader implications for undermining reproductive justice, given the broader long-standing tensions between (pregnant) women's rights and fetal or embryonic protection (Flavin 2008) and the danger that embryonic personhood "may further erode reproductive freedoms . . . for more vulnerable groups" (Cromer 2019, 32). At the same time, a more holistic focus on reproductive rights and reproductive justice necessarily includes the discussion of parentage rights and being able to have and raise one's own children safely and securely (Price 2010; Luna and Luker 2013). To fully address postmodern parentage rights we have to contemplate legal and social relationships to the disembodied embryo as distinct from relationships to fully embodied reproduction. This is necessarily part of a larger conversation about the fragmented, contingent, and uncertain nature of post-IVF maternities.

Acknowledgments

This book has been a long time in the making. My initial thoughts about the topic came out of my dissertation work (2009–2012), but it took another few years for them to develop. After having my first child, I ferociously read more and more sociological and feminist scholarship on motherhood, breast-feeding, and childbirth. These topics were both physically and mentally consuming as I would go on to be pregnant and give birth again, and breast-feed for roughly five to six years of my life across two children. Early stages of the work for this book were especially nurtured by various sessions at the annual Mini-Conference on the Sociology of Reproduction at the meetings of the Eastern Sociological Society. The papers I wrote for these conferences then sat on the back burner for a while, as I was not quite sure what sort of work I was writing. Rosanna Hertz was a catalyst for making me see connections between the various papers and nudging me to submit a book proposal, even though I was not yet sure that I was writing a book. Peggy Nelson turned into a wonderful mentor along the way, giving me patient and constructive feedback every time I managed to email her a chapter or parts of one, as I wrote through the pandemic with little child care for several months. Helpful friends and colleagues in law and political science and several law librarians assisted with legal terms and methods to guide my search for certain parts of my analysis. I learned about "Shepardizing" law, which means to use Shephard's Citations (an authoritative source) to see how and when a case or statute is cited in relation to other legal actions. Helpfully, LexisNexis now has a one-click way of Shepardizing. I also learned that law reviews, no matter how thorough, do not always provide complete data on a subject matter—nor do they often report when a statute was passed, more often noting that something was in effect as the author was writing. This subsequently required a great deal of detective work to find the original effective date of various parentage statutes across the states to track trends over time. This work was mostly done by my wonderful undergraduate research assistant, Christina McCarthy, who has since graduated and started medical school. I cannot thank her enough for the countless hours she spent on LexisNexis and individual state legislature websites, as well as in phone calls with archivists and law librarians, to gather and synthesize much of this data on my behalf. Michele Adams gave time and excitement to the project, reading various chapters that needed another set of eyes on them. I am very grateful to Clare Daniel and the Reproductive Justice Faculty Writing Group for providing accountability and a virtual and mental space to help me commit to my writing every week during the past few semesters. I am indebted to Pat Rafail for his constant support and reminders about my writing process, telling me that every time I feel like I have ripped everything apart, the nice, neat braiding of the pieces back together is usually just around the corner. Thank you to Susan Markens for commenting on the early proposal and to Heather Jacobson for reading a full draft of the manuscript and giving me such kind and constructive comments for revision. Thank you to all the family members, friends, and colleagues who asked me how writing was going and what my book was about over the past several years. Trying to articulate the answers to those questions made the book real and pushed me forward. Thank you to the teachers and staff members at Little Gate and McGehee, who have cared for my girls for years now, and especially for making reopening safe over the past few school years. The in-person schooling and safety protocols in our school community have been invaluable in giving me space to think, read, and write—a necessity that many parents did not have. And finally, thank you to Larry Greil and Julia McQuillan for being my constant mentors for nearly two decades now, encouraging me; believing in me; and eagerly asking about kids, pets, and life along the way.

Notes

Chapter 1   A New Maternity Uncertainty?

1. Biomedically, "infertility" is defined as a year or more with regular, unprotected (heterosexual) sex without conception (American Society for Reproductive Medicine [ASRM] 2008). For critiques of the rigidity and exclusivity of this definition, see Greil and McQuillan (2010) and Johnson et al. (2014).
2. For exceptions see Rothman (1989), Markens (2007), and Teman (2010).
3. Nara Milanich (2017) explores uncertainty in maternity using historical examples such as foundlings and the putting out of children. She argues that the notion of maternity certainty is a social and legal construction. However, I suggest that she is focusing on mothering behavior and the specific relationship of a given mother to a child. In contrast, my focus here is uncertainty as to what constitutes maternity more generally.
4. Lacking such direct observation there might be a case of uncertain maternity, but Stumpf (1986) notes that this probably caused more havoc among the aristocracy, regarding the politics of succession, than among lower classes.

Chapter 2   Conceiving Motherhood and the Repronormative Family

1. At the time, the authors were especially critical of highly medicalized and isolating hospital birth practices in the United States, according to which women and infants were strictly separated in the hours and days

after birth: infants were taken to hospital nurseries and cared for largely by nursing staff members until discharge. Maternal-infant separation and isolation was even more extreme for premature infants.

2. See, for example, the media representations of single men using surrogacy to build families (Johnson 2017c) or recommendations by the American Fertility Society [AFS] Committee on Ethics that assisted reproduction treatments be limited to married heterosexual couples (1986, 1988, 1990, and 1994).

Chapter 3   Losing My Genetics

1. Blackwell was directly critiquing Charles Darwin's and Herbert Spencer's views on evolution and supposedly natural feminine inferiority attributed to women's greater involvement in biological reproduction, which was alleged to limit their mental capacity (Blackwell 1973; Tedesco 1984).

2. Benedek was a student of one of Sigmund Freud's close associates and a major contributor to bringing psychoanalytic thought to the United States in the 1940s.

3. This cure-versus-circumvent approach to infertility has been noted by several reproductive scholars (e.g., Sandelowski [1993], Greil [1991], and Barnes [2014]).

4. The Rh factor in blood was not yet fully understood, which resulted in miscarriages and infant deaths due to discordant Rh status between the pregnant woman and fetus and raised a serious public health concern.

5. Rock would go on to be a coinvestigator with Gregory Pincus in developing the oral contraceptive pill. Menkin was a lab technician who worked on the early IVF experiments. Although Rock is best known for his work on the pill, he spent much of his career researching infertility (Marsh and Ronner 1996).

6. Feminist scholars and activists have had much to say about assisted reproduction (see Lublin [1998] and Thompson [2005] for thorough treatments of this literature). I have chosen to exclude them here for two reasons: I focus on the social worlds that most frequently intersected with reproductive medicine in citations or references to

arguments and scholarship, and these scholars and activitists deserve more adequate consideration than space allows in the current discussion.

7. Watson is best known as one of the discoverers of the double helix structure of DNA—although later reports show how sexism and historical omission marginalized other scientists who significantly contributed to the discovery. His statement on IVF to the House committee was later excerpted in the *Atlantic* for a wider audience.

8. Kass was chairman of the President's Council on Bioethics in the administration of George W. Bush in the early 2000s, when the council specifically addressed IVF and other reproductive technologies (Vastag 2004).

9. Kleegman was the first woman appointed as a professor at the New York University College of Medicine, in 1929 (Marsh and Ronner 1996).

10. This process later fell out of use when physicians found that it made AID less successful in producing pregnancy.

11. Frances Seymour, a New York physician and director of the National Research Foundation for Eugenic Alleviation of Sterility, was one notable exception here (Marsh and Ronner 1996).

12. Initially this was done through laparoscopy (surgery involving a small incision in the abdomen). Later, practitioners switched to transvaginal ultrasound-guided needle aspiration, which dramatically reduced risks to the donor.

13. The rhetoric of a gift is a major frame used in both egg donation and surrogacy (Almeling 2011; Ragone 1999).

14. Notably, the practice of one woman providing an egg and the other gestating was later introduced (and still used) to cement the concept of co-maternity for lesbian couples.

Chapter 4   Contingent Maternities?

A modified version of this chapter was published in the article "Contingent Maternities? Maternal Claims-making in Third-Party Reproduction." It appeared in the journal *Sociology of Health & Illness* in 2017.

1. During my data collection for a prior study on the U.S. fertility industry, several employees from fertility clinics and egg donation

agencies sent me multiple copies of two patient booklets that were being widely used.

2. Of course, in some scenarios the infertility patient might use both a donated embryo and a surrogate. For the purposes of this analysis, I do not focus on these hybrid scenarios. However, one might hypothesize that in such cases, the intended social parents would feel even further removed from their parental status, having neither a genetic nor a gestational connection to the child-to-be.

3. It also invokes ideas from reproductive theories of earlier centuries that women were the incubator or vessel (sometimes referred to as the receptacle of sperm [*receptaculum seminis*]), while men were the true creators of the child (see Guttmacher 1933).

4. Framing surrogacy as a labor of love the surrogate as someone the intended parents cared about also helps avoid connotations of prostitution and baby selling that have come up in commercial surrogacy practices (Berend 2016; Jacobson 2016; Markens 2007; Ragone 1999).

5. There is another scenario, which I do not address here: when a patient uses an embryo created from donor gametes. This scenario does not have the same issues because this type of embryo is no longer a conjugal embryo. The anonymous donors usually do not know one another and are not in a social or legal relationship with one another.

Chapter 5   Designating Maternity

1. In that case, an ex-husband claimed his former spouse was not a natural mother to their children because she had used donor eggs to conceive them.

2. This is the case for both monozygotic (identical) and dizygotic (fraternal) twins, although the former often invoke this sense of wonder to a stronger degree. Twinship research has focused on both the genetic and social and psychological bond of twins, often linking the two (Fortuna, Goldner, and Knafo 2010; Fraley and Tancredy 2012).

3. The media coverage later reported that Robert and Denise were attempting to seek sole custody of Daniel, who by then was approximately 3–4 years old (Chiang 2004). Because the court records are confidential, it is unclear how this final custody battle played out.

4. This has changed due to the Supreme Court decision in *Obergefell v. Hodges* (2015) (Nejaime 2021).

5. Most transracial surrogacy arrangements are also international, with white U.S. intended parents. The surrogacy literature indicates that most domestic U.S. surrogacy arrangements tend to involve racial concordance between both surrogates and intended parents (Jacobson 2016; Ziff 2017).

6. Anna Johnson was ultimately denied legal maternity or visitation rights.

7. I am not suggesting the case was decided incorrectly. I think that procreative intent is a highly useful framework for addressing fragmented or nonbiological parentage. But this points to the issue of all other things being equal, which they usually are not.

8. The reader cannot know what Donna Fasano was thinking about the situation. Nor does Donna have any responsibility for the racialized media framing. At the same time, I think we have to acknowledge that cultural sympathies, expressed through the media coverage, decidedly favored Donna over Deborah Perry-Rogers as the distraught mother of the two boys.

9. A 2007 sperm mix-up case in Oregon supports this possibility. In that case, a judge ruled that a man whose sperm was accidentally used for a patient other than his fiancée had no right to request a paternity test, as the patient was married and her husband was the presumed legal father (Associated Press 2007).

Chapter 6 Adopting or Resisting New Maternities?

1. The ULC has existed since 1892. Its mission, according to the commission, is to provide "states with non-partisan, well-conceived and well-drafted legislation that brings clarity and stability to critical areas of state statutory law" (ULC 2012).

2. As of spring 2021, no other states had enacted such legislation.

3. The Baby M case involved a traditional surrogacy arrangement between MaryBeth Whitehead and Betsy and William Stern in 1985 in New Jersey. After giving birth, MaryBeth had a change of heart and sought to keep the baby. A lower court ruled against her, arguing that

she had relinquished her maternal rights in the initial contract. She appealed, and the Supreme Court of New Jersey invalidated the surrogacy contract but still gave custody to the Sterns.

4. This basic definition of maternity is intriguing because the legal term "preponderance of evidence" simply means that something is more likely than not. In other words, maternity, as defined generally under Louisiana law, does not require establishing absolute certainty.

5. In 2014, he was awarded the Arnold P. Gold Foundation Humanism in Medicine Award from the ASRM. This award goes to practicing physicians who have "demonstrated the ideals of compassionate and respectful care for a patient's physical and emotional well-being" (ASRM 2021).

6. Many would disagree with Krentel's creative interpretation that *Roe v. Wade* created 'property' rights for the pregnant woman over the embryo or fetus: the Supreme Court held that abortion decisions fell within the 'zone of privacy' like contraception and other familial or reproductive decisions. Was he being polemic to gain the moral upper hand?

7. This organization opposed bills in 2013, 2014, and 2016, aiming to defeat them by centering the arguments on the politics of life frame, which appeared prominently in the 1986 Human Embryo Act. They succeeded in securing the governor's veto in 2013 and 2014 but not in 2016, after a change in administration.

8. In other words, that would formally classify it as a "subject of rights and duties" (Hof Wallace 2018, 408). This is not the same as classifying the embryo as a 'natural person,' which would grant it full personhood. In Louisiana law, natural personality is still reserved for the period from live birth to death.

9. They were both listed as "witnesses" and "proponents" in the committee hearing minutes (SB 701 1986b).

10. All the groups he referred to by name in his veto message were either pro-life or explicitly critical of assisted reproduction: the Louisiana Family Forum, Louisiana Conference of Catholic Bishops, Hippocratic Resource, Bioethics Defense Fund, and Center for Bioethics and Culture Network.

11. If the intended parents divorced or annulled their marriage before the embryo transfer procedure, the gestational surrogacy contract was considered void.

12. This had to be obtained within 300 days of the embryo transfer procedure. An average pregnancy is forty weeks (280 days).
13. I interpret the use of possessive language like "our," "my," and "their" as referring to belonging and inclusion in a family group. Such language asserts familial membership and, by extension, relational rights and responsibilities.

Chapter 7   Concluding Thoughts

1. A polyamorous relationship involving three people—a play on "couple."

References

Advance Staff Report. 1999. "2 Moms Ensnared in Embryo Mixup." *Staten Island Advance* March 30.

Agigian, Amy C. 2004. *Baby Steps: How Lesbian Alternative Insemination Is Changing the World*. Middletown, CT: Wesleyan University Press.

Algero, Mary Garvey. 2005. "The Sources of Law and the Value of Precedent: A Comparative and Empirical Study of a Civil Law State in a Common Law Nation." *Louisiana Law Review* 65 (2): 775–822.

Allen, Anita. 1991. "The Black Surrogate Mother." *Harvard Blackletter Journal* 8: 17–32.

Almeling, Rene. 2011. *Sex Cells: The Medical Market for Eggs and Sperm*. Berkeley: University of California Press.

Almeling, Rene, and Miranda Waggoner. 2013. "More and Less than Equal: How Men Factor into the Reproductive Equation." *Gender & Society* 27 (6): 821–842.

American Fertility Society (AFS). 1984. "Ethical Statement on In Vitro Fertilization." *Fertility and Sterility* 41 (1): 12.

———. 1993. "Guidelines for Oocyte Donation." *Fertility and Sterility* 59 (2, supp. 1): 5S-7S.

AFS Committee on Ethics. 1986. "Ethical Considerations of the New Reproductive Technologies." *Fertility and Sterility* 46 (3, supp. 1): iS–94S.

———. 1988. "Ethical Considerations of the New Reproductive Technologies." *Fertility and Sterility* 49 (2, supp. 1): iiiS–7S.

———. 1990. "Ethical Considerations of the New Reproductive Technologies." *Fertility and Sterility* 53 (6, supp. 1): iS–109S.

———. 1994. "Ethical Considerations of Assisted Reproductive Technologies." *Fertility and Sterility* 62 (5, supp. 1): iS–125S.American Pregnancy

Association. 2021. "Nesting during Pregnancy." Retrieved February 2022. https://americanpregnancy.org/healthy-pregnancy/pregnancy-health-wellness/nesting-during-pregnancy/.

American Society for Reproductive Medicine (ASRM). 2008. "Definitions of Infertility and Recurrent Pregnancy Loss." *Fertility and Sterility* 90 (5, supp. 3): S60.

———. 2011. *Assisted Reproductive Technology: A Guide for Patients.* Retrieved January 2013. http://asrm.org/FactSheetsandBooklets/

———. 2012a. *Third Party Reproduction: A Guide for Patients.* Retrieved January 2013. http://asrm.org/FactSheetsandBooklets/

———. 2012b. "Fact Sheet: Embryo Donation." Retrieved January 2013. http://www.reproductivefacts.org/ FactSheetsandBooklets/

———. 2016. "Vision of ASRM." Retrieved January 2016. https://www.asrm.org/about/.

———. 2021. "ASRM Scientific Congress Endowed Awards." Retrieved April 2021. https://www.asrm.org/resources/research-grants-and-awards/asrm-scientific-congress-endowed-awards.

ASRM Ethics Committee. 2006a. "Access to Fertility Treatment by Gays, Lesbians, and Unmarried Persons." *Fertility and Sterility* 86: 1333–1335.

———. 2006b. "Disclosure of Medical Errors Involving Gametes and Embryos." *Fertility and Sterility* 86 (3): 513–515.

———. 2011. "Disclosure of Medical Errors Involving Gametes and Embryos." *Fertility and Sterility* 96 (6): 1312–1314.

———. 2016. "Disclosure of Medical Errors Involving Gametes and Embryos: An Ethics Committee Opinion." *Fertility and Sterility* 106 (1): 59–63.

Andersen, Margaret L. 1991. "Feminism and the American Family Ideal." *Journal of Comparative Family Studies* 22 (2): 235–246.

Anderson, Kermyt G. 2006. "How Well Does Paternity Confidence Match Actual Paternity? Evidence from Worldwide Nonpaternity Rates." *Current Anthropology* 47 (3): 513–520.

Anderson, Linda S. 2009. "Adding Players to the Game: Parentage Determinations When Assisted Reproductive Technology Is Used to Create Families." *Arkansas Law Review* 62: 29–56.

Andrews, Kenneth T., and Bob Edwards. 2004. "Advocacy Organizations in the US Political Process." *Annual Review of Sociology* 30: 479–506.

Andrews, Lori. 1986a. "The Legal Status of the Embryo." *Loyola Law Review* 32 (2): 357–410.

———. 1986b. "My Body, My Property." *Hastings Center Report* 16 (5): 28–38.

Anonymous. 1939. "Editorial: Artificial Insemination and Illegitimacy." *Journal of the American Medical Association* 112 (18): 1832–1833.

Anonymous. 2009. "Ohio Couple Giving Up Baby After Mixup." *Bennington Banner*, September 23.

Arena, Salvatore. 1999a. "Baby Gets New Parents: Judge OK's Swap in Embryo Mixup." *New York Daily News*, June 8.

———. 1999b. "Test-Tube Twins Apart on B'Day." *New York Daily News*, December 30.

Arendell, Terry. 2000. "Conceiving and Investigating Motherhood: The Decade's Scholarship." *Journal of Marriage and Family* 62 (4): 1192–1207.

Arny, Margaret, and John R. Quagliarello. 1987. "History of Artificial Insemination: A Tribute to Sophia Kleegman, M.D." *Seminars in Reproductive Endocrinology* 5 (1): 1–3.

Associated Press. 2007. "Judge Rules against Oregon Man in Sperm Mix-Up." *Seattle Times*, April 17. Retrieved February 2021 https://www.seattletimes.com/seattle-news/judge-rules-against-oregon-man-in-sperm-mix-up/.

Baker, Maureen. 2005. "Medically Assisted Conception: Revolutionizing Family or Perpetuating a Nuclear and Gendered Model?" *Journal of Comparative Family Studies* 36 (4): 521–543.

Barad, David H., and Brian L. Cohen. 1996. "Oocyte Donation Program at Montefiore Medical Center, Albert Einstein College of Medicine, Bronx, New York." In *New Ways of Making Babies: The Case of Egg Donation*, edited by Cynthia B. Cohen, 15–28. Bloomington, IN: Indiana University Press.

Barnes, Liberty Walther. 2014. *Conceiving Masculinity: Male Infertility, Medicine, and Identity*. Philadelphia, PA: Temple University Press.

Beardsley, Grant S. 1940. "Artificial Cross Insemination." *Western Journal of Surgery, Obstetrics, and Gynecology* 48: 94–100.

Becker, Gay. 2000. *The Elusive Embryo: How Men and Women Approach the New Reproductive Technologies*. Berkeley: University of California Press.

———. 2002. "Deciding Whether to Tell Children about Donor Insemination: An Unresolved Question in the United States." In *Infertility around the Globe: New Thinking in Childlessness, Gender, and Reproductive Technologies*, edited by Marcia Inhorn and Frank van Balen, 119–133. Berkeley: University of California Press.

Bell, Ann V. 2014. *Misconception: Social Class and Infertility in America.* New Brunswick, NJ: Rutgers University Press.

———. 2019. "'Trying to Have Your Own First; It's What You Do': The Relationship between Adoption and Medicalized Infertility." *Qualitative Sociology* 42(3): 479–498.

Bender, Leslie. 2006. "'To Err Is Human' ART Mix-Ups: A Labor-Based, Relational Proposal." *Journal of Gender, Race, and Justice* 9 (3): 443–508.

Benedek, Therese. 1960. "The Organization of the Reproductive Drive." *International Journal of Psycho-Analysis* 41: 1–15.

Berend, Zsuzsa. 2016. *The Online World of Surrogacy.* New York: Berghahn Books.

Berend, Zsuzsa, and Corinna Sabrina Guerzoni. 2019. "Reshaping Relatedness? The Case of US Surrogacy." *Antropologia* 6 (2): 83–99.

Berg, Jessica. 2005. "Owning Persons: The Application of Property Theory to Embryos and Fetuses." *Wake Forest Law Review* 40 (1): 159–220.

Bernard, Jessie. 1974. *The Future of Motherhood.* New York: Penguin Books.

———. 1981. "The Good-Provider Role: Its Rise and Fall." *American Psychologist* 36 (1): 1–12.

Bernstein, Gaia. 2002. "The Socio-Legal Acceptance of New Technologies: A Close Look at Artificial Insemination." *Washington Law Review* 77: 1035–1120.

Best, Joel. 1987. "Rhetoric in Claims-Making: Constructing the Missing Children Problem." *Social Problems* 34 (2): 101–121.

Birrittieri, Cara, Mary M. Fusillo, and Georgia Witkin. n.d. *Oocyte Donation.* Freedom Fertility Pharmacy.

Blackwell, Antoinette Brown. 1973. "Sex and Evolution." In *The Feminist Papers: From Adams to de Beauvoir*, edited by Alice Rossi, 356–377. New York: Columbia University Press.

Bloomberg. 2022. "Company Profiles: Organon Pharmaceuticals USA, Inc." Retrieved August 2022 https://www.bloomberg.com/profile/company/0008668D:US

Blumberg, Grace Ganz. 1984. "Legal Issues in Nonsurgical Human Ovum Transfer." *Journal of the American Medical Association* 251 (9): 1178–1181.

Blumer, Herbert. 1969. *Symbolic Interactionism: Perspective and Method.* Berkeley, CA: University of California Press.

Borkan, Jeffrey. 1999. "Immersion/Crystallization." In *Doing Qualitative Research*, 2nd ed., edited by Benjamin Crabtree and William Miller, 179–194. Thousand Oaks, CA: Sage.

Braverman, Andrea Mechanik. 2010. "How the Internet Is Reshaping Assisted Reproduction: From Donor Offspring Registries to Direct-to-Consumer Genetic Testing." *Minnesota Journal of Law, Science, and Technology* 11 (2): 477–496.

Braverman, Andrea Mechanik, and the Ovum Donor Task Force of the Psychological Special Interests Group of the American Fertility Society. 1993. "Survey Results on the Current Practice of Ovum Donation." *Fertility and Sterility* 59 (6): 1216–1220.

Bridges, Tyler. 2020. "Joe Biden Is Buying Ads in Ruby Red Louisiana. But Don't Expect Him to Win on Nov. 3." *Advocate*, October 26. Retrieved March 2021. https://www.theadvocate.com/baton_rouge/news/politics/elections/article_64114b26-17bf-11eb-95b7-d3efe2441ea6.html.

Broad, Kevin D., James P. Curley, and Eric B. Keverne. 2006. "Mother-Infant Bonding and the Evolution of Mammalian Social Relationships." *Philosophical Transactions: Biological Sciences* 361 (1476): 2199–2214.

Brumberg, Joan Jacobs. 1984. "'Ruined' Girls: Changing Community Responses to Illegitimacy in Upstate New York, 1890–1920." *Journal of Social History* 18 (2): 247–272.

Buster, John. 1998. "Historical Evolution of Oocyte and Embryo Donation as a Treatment for Intractable Infertility." In *Principles of Oocyte and Embryo Donation*, edited by Mark V. Sauer, 1–10. New York: Springer.

Bustillo, Maria, John E. Buster, Sydlee Cohen, Ian H. Thorneycroft, James A. Simon, Stephen P. Boyers, John R. Marshall, Randolph W. Seed, John A. Louw, and Richard G. Seed. 1984. "Nonsurgical Ovum Transfer as a Treatment in Infertile Women." *Journal of the American Medical Association* 251 (9): 1171–1173.

Buxton, C. Lee, ed. 1958. "Current Reviews: Artificial Insemination: Genetic, Legal, and Ethical Implications: A Symposium." *Fertility and Sterility* 9 (4): 368–375.

Cahill, Lisa Sowle. 1986. "In Vitro Fertilization: Ethical Issues in Judaeo-Christian Perspective." *Loyola Law Review* 32 (2): 337–356.

Cahn, Naomi. 2009. *Test Tube Families: Why the Fertility Market Needs Legal Regulation.* New York: New York University Press.

———. 2013. *The New Kinship: Constructing Donor-Conceived Families.* New York: New York University Press.

Cahn, Naomi, and June Carbone. 2010. *Red Families v. Blue Families: Legal Polarization and the Creation of Culture.* New York: Oxford University Press.

California Family Code. 2020. §7613. "Establishing Parent and Child Relationship." Retrieved August 2022. https://leginfo.legislature.ca.gov/faces/codes_displaySection.xhtml?lawCode=FAM&sectionNum=7613.

Capron, Alexander M. 1983. "Looking back at the President's Commission." *Hastings Center Report* 13 (5): 7–10.

Centers for Disease Control and Prevention [CDC]. 2022. "ART Success Rates." Retrieved August 2022. https://www.cdc.gov/art/artdata/index.html.

Centers for Disease Control and Prevention [CDC], American Society for Reproductive Medicine [ASRM], and Society for Assisted Reproductive Technology [SART]. 2007. *2005 Assisted Reproductive Technology Success Rates: National Summary and Fertility Clinic Reports.* Atlanta, GA: CDC.

———. 2008. *2006 Assisted Reproductive Technology Success Rates: National Summary and Fertility Clinic Reports.* Atlanta: CDC.

———. 2009. *2007 Assisted Reproductive Technology Success Rates: National Summary and Fertility Clinic Reports.* Atlanta: CDC.

———. 2010. *2008 Assisted Reproductive Technology Success Rates: National Summary and Fertility Clinic Reports.* Atlanta: CDC.

———. 2011. *2009 Assisted Reproductive Technology Success Rates: National Summary and Fertility Clinic Reports.* Atlanta: CDC.

———. 2012. *2010 Assisted Reproductive Technology Success Rates: National Summary and Fertility Clinic Reports.* Atlanta: CDC.

———. 2013. *2011 Assisted Reproductive Technology Success Rates: National Summary and Fertility Clinic Reports*. Atlanta: CDC.

———. 2014. *2012 Assisted Reproductive Technology Success Rates: National Summary and Fertility Clinic Reports*. Atlanta: CDC.

———. 2015. *2013 Assisted Reproductive Technology Success Rates: National Summary and Fertility Clinic Reports*. Atlanta: CDC.

———. 2016. *2014 Assisted Reproductive Technology Success Rates: National Summary and Fertility Clinic Reports*. Atlanta: CDC.

———. 2017. *2015 Assisted Reproductive Technology Success Rates: National Summary and Fertility Clinic Reports*. Atlanta: CDC.

———. 2018. *2016 Assisted Reproductive Technology Success Rates: National Summary and Fertility Clinic Reports*. Atlanta: CDC.

Cherlin, Andrew. 1978. "Remarriage as an Incomplete Institution." *American Journal of Sociology* 84(3): 634–650.

———. 2004. "The Deinstitutionalization of American Marriage." *Journal of Marriage and Family* 66 (4): 848–861.

Chiang, Harriet. 2004. "Mom Awarded $1 Million Over Embryo Mixup." *San Francisco Chronicle*, August 4.

Child Welfare Information Gateway. 2021. "Consent to Adoption." Retrieved March 2022. https://www.childwelfare.gov/topics/systemwide/laws -policies/statutes/consent.

Chodorow, Nancy. 1978. *The Reproduction of Mothering: Psychoanalysis and the Sociology of Gender*. Berkeley: University of California Press.

City News Service. 2021. "Judge Rules in Sofia Vergara's Favor in Frozen Pre-Embryo Lawsuit." NBC, February 5. Retrieved April 2021. https:// www.nbclosangeles.com/news/local/sofia-vergaras-favor-frozen-embryo -lawsuit/2519380/.

Clarke, Adele. 1998. *Disciplining Reproduction: Modernity, American Life Sciences, and the Problems of Sex*. Berkeley, CA: University of California Press.

Clarke, Adele, and Susan Leigh Star. 2008. "The Social Worlds Framework: A Theory/Methods Package." In *The Handbook of Science and Technology Studies*, 3rd ed., edited by Edward Hackett, Olga Ansterdamska, Michael Lynch, and Judy Wajcman, 113–137. Cambridge, MA: MIT Press.

Cohen, Cynthia B. 1996. Introduction to *New Ways of Making Babies: The Case of Egg Donation*, edited by Cynthia B. Cohen, xi–xix. Bloomington: Indiana University Press.

Colen, Shellee. 1995. "'Like a Mother to Them': Stratified Reproduction and West Indian Childcare Workers and Employers in New York." In *Conceiving the New World Order: The Global Politics of Reproduction*, edited by Faye Ginsburg and Rayna Rapp, 78–102. Berkeley: University of California Press.

Collier, Jane, Michelle Z. Rosaldo, and Sylvia Yanagisako. 1992. "Is There a Family? New Anthropological Views." In *Rethinking the Family: Some Feminist Questions*, edited by Barrie Thorne and Marilyn Yalom, 31–48. Boston: Northeastern University Press.

Congregation for the Doctrine of the Faith. 1987. "Instruction on Respect for Human Life in its Origins and on the Dignity of Procreation: Replies to Certain Questions of the Day." Retrieved August 2022. https://www.vatican.va/roman_curia/congregations/cfaith/documents/rc_con_cfaith_doc_19870222_respect-for-human-life_en.html

Conrad, Peter. 1992. "Medicalization and Social Control." *Annual Review of Sociology* 18: 209–232.

Conrad, Peter, and Valerie Leiter. 2004. "Medicalization, Markets, and Consumers." *Journal of Health and Social Behavior* 45 (Extra Issue): 158–176.

Conte, Ronald L., Jr. 2018. "Address of Pope Pius XII on Marriage, Fertility, and Ethics: Translation and Commentary." Retrieved August 2022. http://www.catechism.cc/articles/second-world-congress-fertility-sterility.html

Coulam, Carolyn. 1984. "Editor's Corner: Freezing Embryos." *Fertility and Sterility* 42 (2): 184–186.

Crockin, Susan L., and Howard W. Jones Jr. 2010. *Legal Conceptions: The Evolving Law and Policy of Assisted Reproductive Technologies*. Baltimore, MD: Johns Hopkins University Press.

Cromer, Risa. 2019. "Racial Politics of Frozen Embryo Personhood in the US Antiabortion Movement." *Transforming Anthropology* 27 (1): 22–36.

D'Alton-Harrison, Rita. 2014. "Mater Semper Incertus Est: Who's Your Mummy?" *Medical Law Review* 22 (3): 357–383.

Daniels, Cynthia, and Janet Golden. 2004. "Procreative Compounds: Popular Eugenics, Artificial Insemination, and the Rise of the American Sperm Banking Industry." *Journal of Social History* 38 (1): 5–27.

Davis, M. Edward. 1956. "Editorial: Statement of the American Society for the Study of Sterility Approving Donor Insemination." *Fertility and Sterility* 7(2): 101–102.

DeCherney, Alan H. 1983. "Editor's Corner: Doctored Babies." *Fertility and Sterility* 40 (6): 724–727.

Delaney, Carol. 1986. "The Meaning of Paternity and the Virgin Birth Debate." *Man* 21 (3): 494–513.

Dellenbach, Pierre, Israel Nisand, Laurence Moreau, Brigitte Feger, Claude Plumere, and Pierre Gerlinger. 1985. "Transvaginal Sonographically Controlled Follicle Puncture for Oocyte Retrieval." *Fertility and Sterility* 44(5): 656.

Deomampo, Daisy. 2019. "Racialized Commodities: Race and Value in Human Egg Donation." *Medical Anthropology* 38 (7): 620–633.

Deutsch, Helene. 1991. *Psychoanalysis of the Sexual Functions of Women.* Edited by Paul Roazen. New York: Karnac Books.

Dickey, Richard P. 1986. "The Medical Status of the Embryo." *Loyola Law Review* 32 (2): 317–336.

Dickey, Richard P., and Clyde H. Dorr. 1969. "Oral Contraceptives: Selection of the Proper Pill." *Obstetrics and Gynecology* 33 (2): 273–287.

Dickey, Richard P., Steven N. Taylor, David N. Curole, and Brenda L. Bordson. 1984. "The First In Vitro Fertilization Pregnancy in Louisiana." *Journal of the Louisiana State Medical Society* 136 (2):11–13.

Dickey, Richard P., Steven N. Taylor, David N. Curole, Phillip H. Rye, and Terry T. Olar. 1995. "To the Editor: The Passage of Florida's Statute on Assisted Reproductive Technology." *Obstetrics and Gynecology* 85 (3): 480–481.

Dodd, Jodie, and Caroline Crowther. 2004. "Multifetal Pregnancy Reduction of Triplet and Higher-Order Multiple Pregnancies to Twins." *Fertility and Sterility* 81 (5): 1420–1422.

Dolgin, Janet L. 1997. *Defining the Family: Law, Technology, and Reproduction in an Uneasy Age.* New York: New York University Press.

————. 2000. "Choice, Tradition, and the New Genetics: The Fragmentation of the Ideology of Family." *Connecticut Law Review* 32: 523–566.

Dolinsky, Harriet. 2009. "Emotional Aspects and Issues to Consider
When Deciding to Pursue Third Party Reproduction." Retrieved
October 2016. www.resolve.org/family-building-options/donor-options
/emotional-aspects-and-issues-to-consider-when-deciding-to-pursue
-third-party-reproduction.html

Doody, Kathleen, and Mark Sauer. 2000. *Oocyte Donation: Patient Guide.*
West Orange, New Jersey: Organon Inc.

Doornbos v. Doornbos. 1956. 12 Ill. App.2d 473.

Dow, Dawn Marie 2016. "Integrated Motherhood: Beyond Hegemonic
Ideologies of Motherhood." *Journal of Marriage and Family* 78(1):
180–196.

Dreyfus, Souad. n.d. "Choosing Between Egg Donor and Surrogate."
Retrieved October 2016. http://www.resolve.org/family-building
-options/choosing-between-egg-donor-and-surrogate.html

Duka, Walter E., and Alan H. DeCherney. 1994. *From the Beginning:
A History of the American Fertility Society 1944–1994.* Birmingham, AL:
American Fertility Society.

Dye, Nancy Schrom.1980. "History of Childbirth in America." *Signs* 6 (1):
97–108.

Earle, Sarah. 2003. "Bumps and Boobs: Fatness and Women's Experiences
of Pregnancy." *Women's Studies International Forum* 26 (3): 245–252.

Engels, Frederick. [2001]. *The Origin of the Family, Private Property, and the
State.* Edited with an Introduction by Eleanor Burke Leacock. New
York: International Publishers.

Englert, Yvon, Serena Emiliani, Philippe Revelard, Fabienne Devreker,
Chantal Laruelle, and Anne Delbaere. 2004. "Sperm and Oocyte
Donation: Gamete Donation Issues." *International Congress Series* 1266:
303–310.Ethics Advisory Board. 1979. "Report and Conclusions: HEW
Support of Research Involving Human In Vitro Fertilization and
Embryo Transfer." Washington: Department of Health, Education,
and Welfare.

Eyer, Diane E. 1994. "Mother-Infant Bonding: A Scientific Fiction."
Human Nature 5 (1): 69–94.

Eyer, Katie. 2014. "Constitutional Colorblindness and the Family." *University of Pennsylvania Law Review* 162 (3): 537–604.

Feldman, Jamie. 2020. "This Throuple Made History with Their First Child. Here's What Their Lives Are Like." HuffPost Personal. Retrieved January 2021. https://www.huffpost.com/entry/poly -relationship-adoption-embryo-surr.

Fessler, Ann. 2006. *The Girls Who Went Away: The Hidden History of Women Who Surrendered Children for Adoption in the Decades before Roe v. Wade.* New York: Penguin Books.

Fineman, Martha. 1993. "Our Sacred Institution: The Ideal of the Family in American Law and Society." *Utah Law Review* 387–405.

Finer, Lawrence B., and Mia R. Zolna. 2016. "Declines in Unintended Pregnancy in the United States, 2008–2011." *New England Journal of Medicine* 374 (9):843–852.

Flavin, Jeanne. 2008. *Our Bodies, Our Crimes: The Policing of Women's Reproduction in America.* New York: New York University Press.

Flexner, Eleanor. 1975. *Century of Struggle: The Women's Rights Movement in the United States.* Cambridge, MA: Harvard University Press.

Folsome, Clair E. 1943. "The Status of Artificial Insemination: A Critical Review." *American Journal of Obstetrics & Gynecology* 45 (6): 915–927.

Foote, Jennifer L. 1999. "What's Best for Babies Switched at Birth—The Role of the Court, Rights of Non-Biological Parents, and Mandatory Mediation of the Custodial Agreements." *Whittier Law Review* 21: 315–354.

Fortuna, Keren, Ira Goldner, and Ariel Knafo. 2010. "Twin Relationships: A Comparison across Monozygotic Twins, Dizygotic Twins, and Nontwin Siblings in Early Childhood." *Family Science* 1 (3): 205–211.

Fox, Dov. 2019. *Birth Rights and Wrongs: How Medicine and Technology Are Remaking Reproduction and the Law.* New York: Oxford University Press.

Fraley, R. Chris, and Caroline M. Tancredy. 2012. "Twin and Sibling Attachment in a Nationally Representative Sample." *Personality and Social Psychology Bulletin* 38 (3): 308–316.

Franke, Katherine M. 2001. "Theorizing Yes: An Essay on Feminism, Law, and Desire." *Columbia Law Review* 1010 (1): 181–208.

Franklin, Sarah. 1995. "Postmodern Procreation: A Cultural Account of Assisted Reproduction." In *Conceiving the New World Order: The Global Politics of Reproduction*, edited by Faye Ginsburg and Rayna Rapp, 323–345. Berkeley: University of California Press.

———. 2013. *Biological Relatives: IVF, Stem Cells, and the Future of Kinship*. Durham, NC: Duke University Press.

Freedom Fertility Pharmacy. 2022. "About Freedom Fertility." Retrieved August 2022. https://www.freedomfertility.com/about-us/

Freeman, Andrea. 2020. *Skimmed: Breastfeeding, Race, and Injustice*. Stanford, CA: Stanford University Press.

Gannon, Genevieve. 2020. "Giving Birth to Other Parents' Children." *Australian Women's Weekly*. Retrieved February 19, 2021. https://www.nowtolove.com.au/news/international-news/ivf-babies-swapped-at-birth-62641.

"Genetic Engineering in Man: Ethical Considerations." 1972. *Journal of the American Medical Association* 220 (5): 721.

Gleicher, Norbert. 1984. "Editor's Corner: The Fetus Is a Graft, Both Biologically and Legally." *Fertility and Sterility* 42 (6): 824–825.

Glenn, Evelyn Nakano, Grace Chang, and Linda Rennie Forcey, eds. 1994. *Mothering: Ideology, Experience, and Agency*. New York: Routledge.

Goffman, Erving. 1963. *Stigma: Notes on the Management of a Spoiled Identity*. New York: Simon and Schuster.

Gordon, Linda. 1976. *Woman's Body, Woman's Right: A Social History of Birth Control in America*. New York: Viking Press.

Gorrill, Marsha. 1998. "Selection and Screening of Potential Oocyte Donors." In *Principles of Oocyte and Embryo Donation*, edited by Mark V. Sauer, 35–52. New York: Springer.

Gotanda, Neil. 1995. "A Critique of 'Our Constitution Is Color-Blind.'" In *Critical Race Theory: The Key Writings That Informed the Movement*, edited by Kimberle Crenshaw, Neil Gotanda, Gary Peller, and Kendall Thomas, 257–275. New York: New Press.

Greenhalgh, Trisha, and Richard Peacock. 2005. "Effectiveness and Efficiency of Search Methods in Systematic Reviews of Complex Evidence: Audit of Primary Sources." *British Medical Journal* 331 (5): 1064–1065.

Greil, Arthur L. 1991. *Not Yet Pregnant: Infertile Couples in Contemporary America*. New Brunswick, NJ: Rutgers University Press.

Greil, Arthur L., and Julia McQuillan. 2010. "Trying Times: Medicalization, Intent, and Ambiguity in the Definition of Infertility." *Medical Anthropology Quarterly* 24 (2): 137–156.

Griffin, Larry J. 2000. "Southern Distinctiveness, Yet Again, or, Why America Still Needs the South." *Southern Cultures* 6 (3):47–72.

Gross, Don, and Beth J. Harpaz. 1999. "Embryo Doc on Hot Seat over Mixup." *Staten Island Advance* March 31.

Gubrium, Jaber F., and James A. Holstein. 1993. "Family Discourse, Organizational Embeddedness, and Local Enactment." *Journal of Family Issues* 14 (1): 66–81.

Guttmacher, Alan F. 1933. *Life in the Making*. New York: Garden City Publishing.

———. 1942. "The Role of Artificial Insemination in the Treatment of Sterility." *Journal of the American Medical Association* 120 (6): 442–445.

———. 1943. "The Role of Artificial Insemination in the Treatment of Human Sterility." *Bulletin of the New York Academy of Medicine* 19 (8): 573–591.

———. 1954. "Editorial: Artificial Insemination." *Fertility and Sterility* 5 (1): 4–6.

Guttmacher, Alan F., John O. Haman, and John MacLeod. 1950. "The Use of Donors for Artificial Insemination: A Survey of Current Practices." *Fertility and Sterility* 1 (3): 264–270.

Haimes, Erica. 1993a. "Do Clinicians Benefit from Gamete Donor Anonymity?" *Human Reproduction* 8 (9): 1518–1520.

———. 1993b. "Issues of Gender in Gamete Donation." *Social Science & Medicine* 36 (1): 85–93.

Hamilton, Persis Mary. 1971. *Basic Maternity Nursing*. 2nd ed. St. Louis, Mo.: C. V. Mosby.

Harrison, Laura. 2016. *Brown Bodies, White Babies: The Politics of Cross-Racial Surrogacy*. New York: New York University Press.

Hays, Sharon. 1996. *The Cultural Contradictions of Motherhood*. New Haven, CT: Yale University Press.

Heidt-Forsythe, Erin. 2018. *Between Families and Frankenstein: The Politics of Egg Donation in the United States*. Berkeley: University of California Press.

Hequembourg, Amy. 2004. "Unscripted Motherhood: Lesbian Mothers Negotiate Incompletely Institutionalized Family Relationships." *Journal of Personal and Social Relationships* 21 (6): 739–762.

Hertz, Rosanna, and Margaret K. Nelson. 2019. *Random Families: Genetic Strangers, Sperm Donor Siblings, and the Creation of New Kin*. New York: Oxford University Press.

Hertz, Rosanna, Margaret K. Nelson, and Wendy Kramer. 2015. "Gendering Gametes: The Unequal Contributions of Sperm and Egg Donors." *Social Science & Medicine* 147: 10–19.

Hill Collins, Patricia. 1990. *Black Feminist Thought: Knowledge, Consciousness, and the Politics of Empowerment*. New York: Routledge.

Hinson, Diane S. 2011. "State-by-State Surrogacy Law: Actual Practices." *Family Advocate* 34(2): 36–37.

Hinson, Diane S., and Maureen McBrien. 2011. "Surrogacy Across America." *Family Advocate* 34(2): 32–36.

Hof Wallace, Monica. 2018. "A Primer on Natural and Juridical Persons in Louisiana." *Loyola Law Review* 64 (2): 407–421.

Holstein, James A., and Jaber Gubrium. 1999. "What Is Family?" *Marriage and Family Review* 28 (3–4): 3–20.

Holy See. 2018. "Congregation for the Doctrine of the Faith." Retrieved 2018. http://www.vatican.va/roman_curia/congregations/cfaith/index .htm

Hood, John T. 1958. "The History and Development of the Louisiana Code." *Louisiana Law Review* 19 (1): 18–33.

House Bill [HB] 181. 2000a. Legislature of the State of Louisiana, 1st Extraordinary Session.

———. 2000b. Louisiana House of Representatives, House Floor, 1st Extraordinary Session. March 23. Archival Video.

House Bill [HB] 1102. 2016a. Legislature of the State of Louisiana, Regular Session.

———. 2016b. Hearing Before the Louisiana House of Representatives, Committee on Civil Law and Procedure. April 18. Archival Video

(Testimony in support of HB 1102, Professor Andrea Carroll, Louisiana State Law Institute).

———. 2016c. Hearing Before the Louisiana House of Representatives, Committee on Civil Law and Procedure. April 18. Archival Video (Introduction of HB 1102, Representative Stuart Bishop).

———. 2016d. Hearing Before the Louisiana House of Representatives, Committee on Civil Law and Procedure. April 18. Archival Video (Testimony in support of HB 1102, Katherine Smith, individual).

———. 2016e. Hearing Before the Louisiana House of Representatives, Committee on Civil Law and Procedure. April 18. Archival Video (Presenting HB 1102, Representative Lopinto).

———. 2016f. Hearing Before the Louisiana House of Representatives, Committee on Civil Law and Procedure. April 18. Archival Video (Testimony in support of HB 1102, Loren McIntyre, individual).

———. 2016g. Hearing Before the Louisiana State Senate, Committee on Civil Law and Procedure. Archival Video (Testimony in opposition to HB 1102, Gene Mills, President, Louisiana Family Forum).

———. 2016h. Hearing Before the Louisiana State Senate, Committee on Civil Law and Procedure. Archival Video (Discussion of HB 1102, Representative Tanner Magee).

———. 2016i. Hearing Before the Louisiana State Senate, Committee on Judiciary B. May 10. Archival Video (Testimony in support of HB 1102, Katherine Smith, individual).

———. 2016j. Hearing Before the Louisiana State Senate, Committee on Judiciary B. May 10. Archival Video (Testimony in opposition to HB 1102, Alana Newman, Director, Coalition against Reproductive Trafficking).

———. 2016k. Hearing Before the Louisiana State Senate, Committee on Judiciary B. May 10. Archival Video (Testimony in opposition to HB 1102, Charlotte Bergeron, President, Baton Rouge Right to Life).

Human Embryo Act of 1986. Acts 1986, No. 964, §1. (Louisiana Revised Statutes §9:121–133). Retrieved August 2022. https://legis.la.gov/legis/Law.aspx?p=y&d=108438

Hyde, Laurance M. 1984a. "Child Custody in Divorce—Generally." *Juvenile and Family Court Journal* 35: 1–3.

———. 1984b. "Tender Years Doctrine." *Juvenile and Family Court Journal* 35: 5–16.

Ikemoto, Lisa. 1996. "The In/fertile, the Too Fertile and the Dysfertile." *Hastings Law Journal* 47 (4): 1007–1062.

Jacobson, Heather. 2016. *Labor of Love: Gestational Surrogacy and the Work of Making Babies.* New Brunswick, NJ: Rutgers University Press.

———. 2021. "Commercial Surrogacy in the Age of Intensive Mothering." *Current Sociology Monographs* 69 (2): 193–211.

Jennings, Patricia K. 2006. "The Trouble with the Multi-Ethnic Placement Act: An Empirical Look at Transracial Adoption." *Sociological Perspectives* 49 (4): 559–580.

Jeremiah, Emily. 2006. "Motherhood to Mothering and Beyond: Maternity in Recent Feminist Thought." *Journal of the Association for Research on Mothering* 8 (1–2): 21–33.

Jindal, Bobby. 2013. Veto Message from the Louisiana Governor, RE: Senate Bill No. 162 by Senator Gary Smith. June 20.

Johnson, Katherine M. 2012. "Excluding Lesbian and Single Women? An Analysis of U.S. Fertility Clinic Websites." *Women's Studies International Forum* 35 (5): 394–402.

———. 2017a. "My Gametes, My Right? The Politics of Involving Donors' Partners in Egg and Sperm Donation." *Journal of Law and Medical Ethics* 45(4): 621–633.

———. 2017b. "The Price of an Egg: Oocyte Donor Compensation in the US Fertility Industry." *New Genetics and Society* 36 (4): 354–374.

———. 2017c. "Single, Straight, Wants Kids: Media Framing of Single, Heterosexual Fatherhood via Assisted Reproduction." *Journal of Gender Studies* 26 (4): 387–401.

Johnson, Katherine M., Julia McQuillan, Arthur L. Greil, and Karina M. Shreffler. 2014. "Towards a More Inclusive Framework for Understanding Fertility Barriers." In *Reframing Reproduction: Conceiving Gendered Experiences,* edited by Meredith Nash, 23–38. London: Palgrave MacMillan.

Johnson v. Calvert. 1993. 5 Cal.4th 84.

Jones, Ben. 2009. "University of California Settles Missing Embryo Lawsuits." *BioNews,* September 18. Retrieved February 2022. https://www.bionews.org.uk/page_91862.

Jones, Howard W. 1982. "Editor's Corner: The Ethics of In Vitro Fertilization-1982." *Fertility and Sterility* 37 (2): 146–149.

———. 1983. "Editorials: Variations on a Theme." *Journal of the American Medical Association* 250 (16): 2182–2183.

———. 1989. "Editor's Corner: And Just What Is a Pre-Embryo?" *Fertility and Sterility* 52 (2): 189–191.

———. 1990. "Editor's Corner: Cryopreservation and Its Problems." *Fertility and Sterility* 53 (5): 780–784.

Kaebnick, Gregory. 2004. "The Natural Father: Genetic Paternity Testing, Marriage, and Fatherhood." *Cambridge Quarterly of Healthcare Ethics* 13 (1): 49–60.

Kamischke, A., and E. Nieschlag. 1999. "Analysis of Medical Treatment of Male Infertility." *Human Reproduction* 14 (Supp. 1): 1–23.

Karaian, Lara. 2013. "Pregnant Men: Repronormativity, Critical Trans Theory, and the Re(conceiv)ing of Sex and Pregnancy Law." *Social and Legal Studies* 22 (2): 211–230.

Kiss, Leon. 1971. "Babies by Means of In Vitro Fertilization: Unethical Experiments on the Unborn?" *New England Journal of Medicine* 285 (21): 1174–1179.

Kawash, Samira. 2011. "New Directions in Motherhood Studies." *Signs* 36 (4): 969–1003.

Kempers, Roger. 1980. "Letter from the Editor-in-Chief." *Fertility and Sterility* 34(1): 1–2.

Kennard, Elizabeth A. D., Robert Collins, Josef Blankstein, Leslie R. Schover, George Kanoti, Joann Reiss, and Martin M. Quigley. 1989. "A Program for Matched, Anonymous Oocyte Donation." *Fertility and Sterility* 51 (4): 655–660.

Kim, Mimi E. 2020. "The Carceral Creep: Gender-Based Violence, Race, and the Expansion of the Punitive State, 1973–1983." *Social Problems* 67(2):251–269.

Kindregan, Charles P. 2009. "Considering Mom: Maternity and the Model Act Governing Assisted Reproductive Technology." *Journal of Gender, Social Policy, and the Law* 17 (3): 601–626.

Klaus, Marshall H., and John H. Kennell. 1976. *Maternal-Infant Bonding: The Impact of Early Separation or Loss on Family Development.* Saint Louis, Mo: C. V. Mosby.

Kleegman, Sophia J. 1954. "Therapeutic Donor Insemination." *Fertility and Sterility* 5 (1): 7–31.

Klein, Nancy A., Gretchen Sewall, and Michael Soules. 1996. "Donor Oocyte Program at University of Washington Medical Center, Seattle, Washington." In *New Ways of Making Babies: The Case of Egg Donation*, edited by Cynthia B. Cohen, 3–14. Bloomington: Indiana University Press.

Kluchin, Rebecca M. 2011. *Fit to Be Tied: Sterilization and Reproductive Rights in America, 1950–1980.* New Brunswick, NJ: Rutgers University Press.

Krentel, John. 1985. "'Ownership' of the Fertilized Ovum In Vitro: A Hypothetical Case in Louisiana." *Louisiana Bar Journal* 32: 284–290.

———. 1999. "The Louisiana 'Human Embryo' Statute Revisited: Reasonable Recognition and Protection for the In Vitro Fertilized Ovum." *Loyola Law Review* 45 (2): 239–246.

Lauer, Robert H., and Warren H. Handel. 1977. *Social Psychology: The Theory and Application of Symbolic Interactionism.* Boston: Houghton Mifflin.

Laws-King, Andrea, Alan Trounson, Henry Sathananthan, and Ismail Kola.1987. "Fertilization of Human Oocytes by Micro-Injection of a Single Spermatozoon under the Zona Pellucida." *Fertility and Sterility* 48 (4): 637–642.

Lebovic, Dan I., John David Gordon, and Robert N. Taylor. 2014. *Reproductive Endocrinology and Infertility: Handbook for Clinicians.* 2nd ed. Arlington, VA: Scrub Hill Press.

Leeton, John. 2013. *Test Tube Revolution: The Early History of IVF.* Clayton, Victoria, Australia: Monash University Publishing.

Lessor, Roberta. 1993. "All in the Family: Social Processes in Ovarian Egg Donation between Sisters." *Sociology of Health & Illness* 15 (3):393–431.

Lessor, Roberta, NancyAnn Cervantes, Nadine O'Connor, Jose Balmaceda, and Ricardo Asch. 1993. "An Analysis of Social and Psychological Characteristics of Women Volunteering to Become Oocyte Donors." *Fertility and Sterility* 59 (1): 65–71.

Letherby, Gayle. 1999. "Other Than Mother and Mothers as Others: The Experience of Motherhood and Non-Motherhood in Relation to

'Infertility' and 'Involuntary Childlessness.'" *Women's Studies International Forum* 22 (3): 359–372.

Lorber, Judith, and Lisa Jean Moore. 2006. *Gendered Bodies, Feminist Perspectives* New York: Oxford University Press.

Louisiana Civil Code. 2009. Article 184. "Maternity." Retrieved August 2022. http://legis.la.gov/Legis/Law.aspx?d=109079

Louisiana Family Forum. 2022. "Home." Retrieved August 2022. https://www.lafamilyforum.org/

Louisiana Official Revision Comments. 2017. §9:2720.5. "Order Preceding Embryo Transfer." LexisNexis Louisiana Annotated Statutes.

Louisiana Revised Statute. 1986. §9:126. "Ownership." Retrieved August 2022. https://legis.la.gov/legis/Law.aspx?d=108443

Louisiana Revised Statute. 1987. §9:2713. "Contract for Surrogate Motherhood; Nullity." Retrieved August 2022. https://law.justia.com/codes /louisiana/2013/code-revisedstatutes/title-9/rs-9-2713

Louisiana Revised Statute. 2016. §9:2720.13. "Post-Birth Order." Retrieved August 2022. http://legis.la.gov/legis/Law.aspx?d=1015759

Louisiana Revised Statute. 2018. §14:89. "Crime Against Nature." Retrieved August 2022. http://www.legis.la.gov/legis/law.aspx?d =78695

Louisiana Right to Life. 2020. "Our Mission." Retrieved April 2021. https://prolifelouisiana.org/mission.

Lublin, Nancy. 1998. *Pandora's Box: Feminism Confronts Reproductive Technology*. Lanham, MD: Rowman and Littlefield.

Luna, Zakiya, and Kristin Luker. 2013. "Reproductive Justice." *Annual Review of Law and Social Science* 9(1): 327–352.

Lutjen, Peter, Alan Trounson, John Leeton, Jock Findlay, Carl Wood, and Peter Renou. 1984. "The Establishment and Maintenance of Pregnancy Using In Vitro Fertilization and Embryo Donation in a Patient with Primary Ovarian Failure." *Nature* 307: 174–175.Mabry, Cynthia R. 2004. "'Who Is My Real Father?' The Delicate Task of Identifying a Father and Parenting Children Created from an In Vitro Mix-Up." *National Black Law Journal* 18 (1):1–62.

MacDonald, Cameron. 2010. *Shadow Mothers: Nannies, Au Pairs, and the Micropolitics of Mothering*. Berkeley: University of California Press.

Maestripieri, Dario. 2001. "Is There Mother-Infant Bonding in Primates?" *Developmental Review* 21 (1): 93–120.

Mamo, Laura. 2007. *Queering Reproduction: Achieving Pregnancy in the Age of Technoscience*. Durham, NC: Duke University Press.

Markens, Susan. 2007. *Surrogate Motherhood and the Politics of Reproduction*. Berkeley: University of California Press.

Marks, Lara. 1999. "'Not Just a Statistic': The History of USA and UK Policy over Thrombotic Disease and the Oral Contraceptive Pill, 1960s–1970s." *Social Science & Medicine* 49 (9): 1139–1155.

Marsh, Margaret, and Wanda Ronner. 1996. *The Empty Cradle: Infertility in America from Colonial Times to the Present*. Baltimore, MD: Johns Hopkins University Press.

Martin, Emily. 1991. "The Egg and the Sperm: How Science Has Constructed a Romance Based on Stereotypical Male-Female Roles." *Signs* 16 (3): 485–501.

Martin, Lauren Jade. 2009. "Reproductive Tourism in the Age of Globalization." *Globalizations* 6 (2): 249–263.

———. 2015. *Reproductive Tourism in the United States: Creating Family in the Mother Country*. New York: Routledge.

Martin, Patricia Yancey. 2004. "Gender as Social Institution." *Social Forces* 82 (4): 1249–1273.

Marshak, Hilary. 2009. "Donors' Attitudes About Egg Donation." Retrieved October 2016. http://www.resolve.org/family-building -options/donor-options/donors-attitudes-about-egg-donation.html

May, Jeffrey. V., and Kelly. Hanshew. 1990. "Organization of the In Vitro Fertilization and Embryo Transfer Laboratory." In *CRC Handbook of the Laboratory Diagnosis and Treatment of Infertility*, edited by Brooks Keel and Bobby Webster, 291–328. Boca Raton, FL: CRC Press.

McDonald v. McDonald. 1994. 196 A.D.2d 7.

Medical Research International (MRI), Society for Assisted Reproductive Technology (SART), and American Fertility Society (AFS). 1990. "In Vitro Fertilization-Embryo Transfer in the United States: 1988 Results from the IVF-ET Registry." *Fertility and Sterility* 53 (1): 13–20.

Mercer, Ramona T. 2004. "Becoming a Mother versus Maternal Role Attainment." *Journal of Nursing Scholarship* 36 (3): 226–232.

Miall, Charlene, and Karen March. 2003. "A Comparison of Biological and Adoptive Mothers and Fathers: The Relevance of Biological Kinship and Gendered Constructs of Parenthood." *Adoption Quarterly* 6 (4): 7–39.

Michelle, Carolyn. 2006. "Transgressive Technologies? Strategies of Discursive Containment in the Representation and Regulation of Assisted Reproductive Technologies in Aotearoa/New Zealand." *Women's Studies International Forum* 29 (2): 109–124.

Midgley, James. 1992. "Society, Social Policy, and the Ideology of Reaganism." *Journal of Sociology & Social Welfare* 19 (1): 13–28.

Milanich, Nara. 2017. "Certain Mothers, Uncertain Fathers: Placing Assisted Reproductive Technologies in Historical Perspective." In *Reassembling Motherhood: Procreation and Care in a Globalized World*, edited by Yasmine Ergas, Jane Jenson, and Sonya Michel, 17–37. New York: New York University Press.

Miller, Molly. 2010. "Embryo Adoption: The Solution to an Ambiguous Intent Standard." *Minnesota Law Review* 94: 869–895.

Morse, Janice. 1995. "The Significance of Saturation." *Qualitative Health Research* 5 (2): 147–149.

Muzio, Cheryl. 1993. "Lesbian Co-Parenting: On Being/Being with the Invisible (M)other." *Smith College Studies in Social Work* 63 (3): 215–229.

Naples, Nancy A. 2004. "Queer Parenting in the New Millennium." *Gender & Society* 18 (6): 679–684.

Nejaime, Douglas. 2017. "The Nature of Parenthood." *Yale Law Journal* 126 (8): 2260–2381.

———. 2021. "Who Is a Parent?" *Family Advocate* 43 (4): 6–9.

Nelson, Margaret. 2006. "Single Mothers 'Do' Family." *Journal of Marriage and Family* 68 (4): 781–795.

New York Domestic Relations Law. 2021. CH 14, §8:122. "Public Policy." Retrieved August 2022. https://www.nysenate.gov/legislation/laws /DOM/122

Obergefell v. Hodges, 2015. No. 14-556 (U.S. June 26, 2015e).

O'Connor, B. B. 1993. "The Home Birth Movement in the United States." *Journal of Medicine and Philosophy* 18: 147–174.

Ogburn, William F. 1922. *Social Change with Respect to Culture and Original Nature*. New York: B. W. Huebsch.

Ombelet, Willem, and Johan. Van Robays. 2015. "Artificial Insemination History: Hurdles and Milestones." *Facts and Views in Visual OB/GYN* 7 (2): 137–143.

Orde, J. 1922. "Orford v. Orford." In *The Ontario Law Reports: Cases Determined in the Supreme Court of Ontario (Appellate and High Court Divisions), Volume XLIX, 1921,* edited by Edward B. Brown, 15–24. Toronto, CAN: Canada Law Book Company, Limited.

Orford v. Orford, 1921. 58 D.L.R. 251.

Pande, Amrita. 2009. "'It May Be Her Eggs but It's My Blood': Surrogates and Everyday Forms of Kinship in India." *Qualitative Sociology* 32: 379–397.

Parsons, Talcott, and Robert F. Bales. 1956. *Family Socialization and Interaction Process.* Oxon, UK: Routledge.

Perry-Rogers v. Fasano, 2000. 276 A.D.2d 67, 715 N.Y.S.2d 19 (App. Div.).

Perry-Rogers v. Fasano, 2001. 96 N.Y.2d 712; 754 N.E.2d 199; 729 N.Y.S.2d 439; N.Y. LEXIS 1067.

Petchesky, Rosalind P. 1987. "Fetal Images: The Power of Visual Culture in the Politics of Reproduction." *Feminist Studies* 13 (2): 263–292.

Pleck, Joseph. 1998. "American Fathering in Historical Perspective." In *Families in the US: Kinship and Domestic Politics,* edited by Karen V. Hansen and Anita Ilta Garey, 351–362. Philadelphia, PA: Temple University Press.

Portnoy, Louis. 1956. "Artificial Insemination (A.I.D.): Experiences with Its Use in Eighty Barren Marriages." *Fertility and Sterility* 7 (4): 327–340.

Practice Committee of the American Society for Reproductive Medicine and Society for Assisted Reproductive Technology. 2012. "Intracytoplasmic Sperm Injection (ICSI) for Non-Male Factor Infertility: A Committee Opinion." *Fertility and Sterility* 98 (6): 1395–3199.

Price, Kimala. 2010. "What Is Reproductive Justice? How Women of Color Activists Are Redefining the Pro-Choice Paradigm." *Meridians* 10 (2): 42–65.

Purhonen, Maija, Riitta Kilpeläinen-Lees, Ari Pääkkönen, Heidi Yppärilä, Johannes Lehtonen, and Jari Karhu. 2001. "Effects of Maternity on Auditory Event-Related Potentials to Human Sound." *NeuroReport* 12 (13): 2975–2979.

Quigley, Martin M., and Lori B. Andrews. 1984. "Human In Vitro Fertilization and the Law." *Fertility and Sterility* 42 (3): 348–355.

Ragone, Helena. 1999. "The Gift of Life: Surrogate Motherhood, Gamete Donation, and Constructions of Altruism." In *Transformative Motherhood: On Giving and Getting in a Consumer Culture*, edited by Linda Layne, 65–88. New York: New York University Press.

Ramsey, Paul. 1972a. "Shall We 'Reproduce'? I. The Medical Ethics of In Vitro Fertilization." *Journal of the American Medical Association* 220 (10): 1346–1350.

———. 1972b. "Shall We 'Reproduce'? II. Rejoinders and Future Forecast." *Journal of the American Medical Association* 220 (11): 1480–1485.

Research Correlating Committee of the American Society for the Study of Sterility. 1951. "Evaluation of the Barren Marriage." *Fertility and Sterility* 2 (1): 1–14.

RESOLVE: The National Infertility Association (RESOLVE). n.d.a. *Embryo Donation, A Family Building Option: What Recipient Couples Should Know.*

———. n.d.b. *Embryo Donation, A Family Building Option: What Donor Couples Should Know.*

———. 2016a. "About Us." Retrieved October 2016. http://www.resolve.org/about/

———. 2016b. "Embryo Donation." Retrieved October 2016. http://www.resolve.org/archive/about/embryo-donation.html

———. 2016c. "Maggie's Story." Retrieved October 2016. http://www.resolve.org/family-building-options/donor-options/maggie-s-story.html

———. 2016d. "Mary's Story." Retrieved October 2016. http://www.resolve.org/family-building-options/donor-options/mary-s-story.html

———. 2016e. "Surrogacy" Retrieved October 2016. http://www.resolve.org/family-building-options/surrogacy/what-is-surrogacy.html

———. 2016f. "Questions to Ask Series: About Surrogacy Programs." Retrieved October 2016. http://familybuilding.resolve.org/site/DocServer/Surrogacy_Programs.pdf?docID=544

Rich, Adrienne. 1980. "Compulsory Heterosexuality and Lesbian Existence." *Signs* 5 (4): 631–660.

———. 1986. *Of Woman Born: Motherhood as Experience and Institution.* New York: Norton

Robert B. v. Susan B., 2003. 135 Cal. Rptr. 2d 785, 109 Cal. App. 4th 1109 (Ct. App.).

Roberts, John. 1995. "News: US Doctors Accused of Misusing Embryos." *British Medical Journal* 311 (7005): 585.

Roberts, Dorothy. 1997. *Killing the Black Body: Race, Reproduction, and the Meaning of Liberty*. New York: Vintage Books.

Rock, John, and Miriam F. Menkin. 1944. "In Vitro Fertilization and Cleavage of Human Ovarian Eggs." *Science* 100 (2588): 105–107

Roe v. Wade, 1973. 410 U.S. 113, 93 S. Ct. 705, 35 L. Ed. 2d 147.

Rosenwaks, Zev. 1987. "Donor Eggs: Their Application in Modern Reproductive Technologies." *Fertility and Sterility* 47 (6): 895–909

Rothman, Barbara Katz. 1989. *Recreating Motherhood: Ideology and Technology in a Patriarchal Society*. New York: W. W. Norton.

Rudavsky, Shari. 1999. "Separating Spheres: Legal Ideology v. Paternity Testing in Divorce Cases." *Science in Context* 12 (1): 123–138.

Russell, Camisha A. 2018. *The Assisted Reproduction of Race*. Bloomington: Indiana University Press.

Saldana, Johnny. 2009. *The Coding Manual for Qualitative Researchers*. Los Angeles: Sage.

Sandelowski, Margarete. 1993. *With Child in Mind: Studies of the Personal Encounter with Infertility*. Philadelphia: University of Pennsylvania Press.

Sauer, Mark V. 1996. "Oocyte Donation: Reflections on Past Work and Future Directions." *Human Reproduction* 11 (6): 1149–1155.

Sauer, Mark V., and Suzanne Kavic. 2006. "Oocyte and Embryo Donation 2006: Reviewing Two Decades of Innovation and Controversy." *Reproductive BioMedicine Online* 12 (2): 153–162.

Sauer, Mark V., and Richard J. Paulson. 1992. "Understanding the Current Status of Oocyte Donation in the United States: What's Really Going on Out There?" *Fertility and Sterility* 58 (1): 16–18.

Sauer, Mark V., Ingrid Rodi, Michelle Scrooc, Maria Bustillo, and John E. Buster. 1988. "Survey of Attitudes Regarding the Use of Siblings for Gamete Donation." *Fertility and Sterility* 49 (4): 721–722.

Schatkin, Sydney B. 1954. "The Legal Aspect of Artificial Insemination." *Fertility and Sterility* 5 (1): 40–43.

Schlegel, P. N. 2004. "Causes of Azoospermia and Their Management." *Reproduction, Fertility, and Development* 16 (5): 561–572.

Schneider, David M. 1984. *A Critique of the Study of Kinship.* Ann Arbor: University of Michigan Press.

Seashore, R. T. 1938. "Artificial Impregnation." *Minnesota Medicine* 21: 641–644.

Seewer, John. 2009. "Ohio Couple Giving Up Baby after Mixup." Associated Press, September 23.

Seibel, Machelle M., and Susan L. Crockin. 1996. *Family Building through Egg and Sperm Donation: Medical, Legal, and Ethical Issues.* Boston: Jones and Bartlett.

Senate Bill [SB] 701.1986a. Legislature of the State of Louisiana, 12th Regular Session.

———. 1986b. Minutes of the Hearing Before the Louisiana House of Representatives, Committee on Civil Law and Procedure. June 16.

Seymour, Frances, and Alfred Koerner. 1936. "Medicolegal Aspect Artificial Insemination." *Journal of the American Medical Association* 107(19): 1531–1534.

———. 1941. "Artificial Insemination: Present Status in the United States as Shown by a Recent Survey." *Journal of the American Medical Association* 116 (25): 2747–2749

Sherman, Jerome K. 1973. "Synopsis of the Use of Frozen Human Semen since 1964: State of the Art of Human Semen Banking." *Fertility and Sterility* 24 (5): 397–412.

Shields, Frances. 1950. "Artificial Insemination as Related to the Female." *Fertility and Sterility* 1 (3): 271–280.

Simmons, Fred A. 1957. "Role of the Husband in Therapeutic Donor Insemination." *Fertility and Sterility* 8 (6): 547–550.

Simon, Michael S. 1991. "'Honey, I Froze the Kids': *Davis v. Davis* and the Legal Status of Early Embryos." *Loyola University Chicago Law Journal* 23 (1): 131–154.

Singer, Jana. 2006. "Marriage, Biology, and Paternity: The Case for Revitalizing the Marital Presumption." *Maryland Law Review* 65: 246–270.

Smith, Dorothy E. 1993. "The Standard North American Family: SNAF as an Ideological Code." *Journal of Family Issues* 14 (1): 50–65.

Solinger, Ricki. 1994. "Race and 'Value': Black and White Illegitimate Babies, 1945–1965." In *Mothering: Ideology, Experience, and Agency*, edited by Evelyn Nakano Glenn, Grace Chang, and Linda Rennie Forcey, 287–310. New York: Routledge.

Spar, Debra. 2006. *The Baby Business: How Money, Science, and Politics Drive the Commerce of Conception*. Boston: Harvard Business Press.

Stacey, Judith. 1996. *In the Name of The Family: Rethinking Family Values in the Postmodern Age*. Boston: Beacon Press.

Stepita, C. Travers. 1933. "Physiologic Artificial Insemination." *American Journal of Surgery* 21 (3): 450–451.

Strauss, Anselm. 1978. "A Social World Perspective." *Studies in Symbolic Interaction* 1: 119–128.

Strnad v. Strnad, 1948. 78 NYS 2d 390.

Stumpf, Andrea E. 1986. "Redefining Mother: A Legal Matrix for New Reproductive Technologies." *Yale Law Journal* 96 (1): 187–208.

Surrogacy Arrangements Act of 1987. 1987. *Hearings on H.R. 2433 Before the Subcommittee on Transportation, Tourism, and Hazardous Materials of the Committee on Energy and Commerce*, 100th Congress. October 15. (Testimony of Arthur Morrell, Louisiana State representative).

Tarrow, Sydney. 2011. *Power in Movement: Social Movements and Contentious Politics*. 3rd ed. New York: Cambridge University Press.

Taylor, Verta. 1996. *Rock-a-Bye Baby: Feminism, Self-Help, and Post-Partum Depression*. New York: Routledge.

Tedesco, Marie. 1984. "A Feminist Challenge to Darwinism: Antoinette L.B. Blackwell on the Relations of the Sexes in Nature and Society." In *Feminist Visions: Toward a Transformation of the Liberal Arts Curriculum*, edited by Diane L. Fowlkes and Charlotte S. McClure, 53–65. University of Alabama Press.

Teman, Elly. 2010. *Birthing a Mother: The Surrogate Body and the Pregnant Self*. Berkeley: University of California Press.

Thompson, Charis. 2002. "Fertile Ground: Feminists Theorize Infertility." In *Infertility around the Globe: New Thinking in Childlessness, Gender, and Reproductive Technologies*, edited by Marcia Inhorn and Frank van Balen, 52–78. Berkeley: University of California Press.

———. 2005. *Making Parents: The Ontological Choreography of Reproductive Technologies*. Cambridge, MA: MIT Press.

Trounson, Alan. 1986. "Preservation of Human Eggs and Embryos." *Fertility and Sterility* 46 (1): 1–12.

Uniform Law Commission [ULC]. 2012. "About Us." Retrieved October 2020. https://www.uniformlaws.org/aboutulc/overview.

———. 2021a. "Parentage Act (1973)." Retrieved April 2021. https://www.uniformlaws.org/committees/community-home?CommunityKey=10720858-ebe1-4e85-a275-40210e3f3f87.

———. 2021b. "Parentage Act (2002)." Retrieved April 2021. https://www.uniformlaws.org/committees/community-home?CommunityKey=5d5c48d6-623f-4d01-9994-6933ca8af315.

———. 2021c. "2017 Parentage Act." Retrieved April 2021. https://www.uniformlaws.org/committees/community-home?CommunityKey=c4f37d2d-4d20-4be0-8256-22dd73af068f.

Utian, W. H., L. Sheean, J. M. Goldfarb, and R. Kiwi. 1985. "Letter to the Editor: Successful Pregnancy after In Vitro Fertilization and Embryo Transfer from an Infertile Woman to a Surrogate." *New England Journal of Medicine* 313 (21): 1351–1352.

Vastag, Brian. 2004. "Group Calls for Stricter Rules for Assisted Reproduction, Ban of 'Extreme' Technologies." *Journal of the American Medical Association* 291 (19): 2306–2308.

Verbian, Channa. 2006. "White Birth Mothers of Black/White Biracial Children: Addressing Racialized Discourses in Feminist and Multicultural Literature." *Journal of the Association for Research on Mothering* 8 (1–2): 213–222.

Vermont Statutes Annotated. 2017. 15C §709. "Laboratory Error." Retrieved August 2022. https://legislature.vermont.gov/statutes/section/15C/007/00709

Walters, LeRoy. 1983. "Ethical Aspects of Surrogate Embryo Transfer." *Journal of the American Medical Association* 250 (16): 2183–2184.

Watson, James D. 1971. "Moving toward the Clonal Man: Is This What We Want?" *Atlantic*, May. Retrieved January 2020. https://www.theatlantic.com/magazine/archive/1971/05/moving-toward-the-clonal-man/305435/

Weaver, Shannon E., and Marilyn Coleman. 2005. "A Mothering but Not a Mother Role: A Grounded Theory Study of a Nonresidential Stepmother Role." *Journal of Social and Personal Relationships* 22 (4): 477–497.

Wegar, Katarina. 1997. "In Search of 'Bad' Mothers: Social Constructions of Birth and Adoptive Motherhood." *Women's Studies International Forum* 20 (1): 77–86.

———. 1998. "Adoption and Kinship." In *Families in the US: Kinship and Domestic Politics*, edited by Karen V. Hansen and Anita Ilta Garey, 41–54. Philadelphia, PA: Temple University Press.

Weick, Karl E. 1995. *Sensemaking in Organizations*. Thousand Oaks, CA: Sage.

Weisman, Abner I. 1942. "The Selection of Donors for Use in Artificial Insemination." *Western Journal of Surgery, Obstetrics, and Gynecology* 50: 142–144.

Weissman, Anna L. 2017. "Repronormativity and the Reproduction of the Nation-State: The State and Sexuality Collide." *Journal of GLBT Family Studies* 13 (3): 277–305

Weitz, Tracy. 2009. "What Physicians Need to Know about the Legal Status of Abortion in the United States." *Clinical Obstetrics and Gynecology* 52 (2): 130–139.

West, Candace, and Sarah Fenstermaker. 1993. "Power, Inequality, and the Accomplishment of Gender: An Ethnomethodological View." In *Theory on Gender/Feminism on Theory*, edited by Paula England, 151–174]. New York: Walter de Gruyter.

West, Candace, and Don H. Zimmerman. 1987. "Doing Gender." *Gender & Society* 1 (2): 125–151.

Weston, Kath. 1991. *Families We Choose: Lesbians, Gays, Kinship*. New York: Columbia University Press.

Wiessinger, Diane, Diana West, and Teresa Pitman. 2010. *The Womanly Art of Breastfeeding*. 8th ed. New York: Ballantine Books.

Williams, Jamie. 2011. "Myths About Surrogates/Gestational Carriers." Retrieved October 2016 http://www.resolve.org/family-building-options/surrogacy/myths-about-surrogates-gestational-carriers.html

Wilson, J. T. 1914. "Observations upon Young Human Embryos." *Journal of Anatomy and Physiology* 48 (Pt 3): 315–351.

Wimalasundera, R. C. 2010. "Selective Reduction and Termination of Multiple Pregnancies." *Seminars in Fetal and Neonatal Medicine* 15: 327–335.

Wolfberg, Elias. 1999. "NJ Couple Wins Permanent Custody from Island Birth Mother and Husband." *Staten Island Advance*, July 17.

Wong, Sau-Ling C. 1994. "Diverted Mothering: Representations of Caregivers of Color in the Age of Multiculturalism." In *Mothering: Ideology, Experience, and Agency*, edited by Evelyn Nakano Glenn, Grace Chang, and Linda Rennie Forcey, 67–94. New York: Routledge.

Zelizer, Viviana. 1985. *Pricing the Priceless Child: The Changing Social Value of Children*. New York: Basic Books.

———. 2000. "The Purchase of Intimacy." *Law & Social Inquiry* 25 (3): 817–848.

Ziff, Elizabeth. 2017. "The Mommy Deployment: Military Spouses and Surrogacy in the United States." *Sociological Forum* 32 (2): 406–425.

Index

abortion, 45; egg donation in history of, 71, 72, 77; and embryo mix-up cases, 133–134; and family values, 141; and in-vitro fertilization, 55; and politics of life, 57, 133; privacy rights in, 54, 56; and property rights of pregnant woman, 146, 180n6; religious beliefs on, 104; *Roe v. Wade* (1973) case on, 54–55, 56, 57, 140, 146

adoption, 4, 80; birth mother in, 4, 32, 41; of donor-conceived children, 61; in embryo donation, 89, 99, 100, 149, 150; in gestational surrogacy, 155–161; in hierarchy of family-building options, 89; intrauterine, egg donation as, 65; by nonbiological co-mothers, 31–32; patient literature on, 88, 89; race in, 46, 125, 127; sentimental, 46; in sperm donation, 59; state laws on, 142; waiting period for consent to, 32; of young white children, 46

adultery: artificial insemination as, 50, 51, 57–58, 76, 139; in vivo egg donation as, 68

agenda-setting organizations in reproductive medicine, 81, 99

Alabama, 143

Allen, Anita, 127

altruism, gestational surrogacy as, 154

American College of Obstetricians and Gynecologists, 54

American Fertility Society (AFS): on egg donation, 66, 67, 69, 74; on ethics of IVF, 55–56, 66, 146; funding ethics board, 54; on in vitro fertilization, 55–56; Jones role in, 48; and Louisiana legislation, 146, 148; name changes of, 22, 81; publications as research resource, 22, 23, 24; on recipients of fertility services, 85, 176n2; on success of IVF, 48

American Journal of Obstetrics & Gynecology, 23, 49

American Journal of Surgery, 60

American Medical Association, 51

American Pregnancy Association, 29

American Society for Reproductive Medicine (ASRM), 82, 85–87; as agenda-setting organization, 81; on egg donation, 90; on embryo donation, 97, 98; on embryo mix-up cases, 116, 132–133; on gestational surrogacy, 88, 95; norms in literature of, 101; organizational goals of, 81, 85–86; prior names of, 22, 81; publications as research resource, 22, 24, 81; on recipients of fertility services, 85; in social world of reproductive medicine, 19–20

American Society for the Study of Sterility (ASSS), 22, 50, 52, 81

Andersen, Margaret, 39

Anderson, Linda, 18

Andrews, Lori, 148–149

social worlds, 18–21, 35, 44; arena of action
or concern in, 19, 20; discourse in, 18,
19; of law, 19–21, 102; of reproductive
medicine, 19–21, 81, 85, 102
socioeconomic status and infertility
experience, 33
Solinger, Ricki, 41
southern states, 136, 138. *See also*
Louisiana
sperm donation: adoption analogy of,
59; and adoption of donor-conceived
children, 61; as adultery, 50, 51, 57–58,
76, 139; and attachment of donors to
sperm, 76; beliefs on parting with
and receiving sperm, 22; compared to
egg donation, 66–68, 74, 75–78;
consent in, 50, 52, 58, 139; and
deinstitutionalization of family
relationships, 6–7; disclosure to
donor-conceived children on, 64; and
fathering, 44; forgotten man in, 63,
68; friends or relatives as donors in,
63, 70, 78; intent in, 59–60, 120; legal
issues in, 3, 15, 45, 49, 50, 51–52, 58,
135, 139–140, 179n9; legitimacy of
children in, 50, 52, 57, 58, 76, 135, 139;
literature analysis on, 23, 24; medical
response to, 49, 50–51; medical social
control in, 61–64; medical students as
donors in, 62–63, 71; mix-up and use
of wrong sperm in, 108; motivation of
donors in, 45, 67–68; paternity in, 3,
10, 12, 15, 45, 57–58, 60–61, 74, 76,
139–140; physician liability concerns
in, 58, 62; and politics of family, 21,
44, 57, 75–76, 139; primary users of,
165; recommendations for use of, 47;
secrecy and confidentiality in, 8, 13,
15, 45, 63–64, 74, 76; selection of
donors in, 62–63, 75; selection of
recipients in, 61–62; sexual connotations in, 77–78; social propriety of, 59;
state laws on, 3, 15, 52, 135, 139–140
sperm of husband: in AI, 47, 49, 50, 60,
68, 140, 177n10; in gestational

surrogacy, 152–153, 158, 159; in in vivo
fertilization and uterine lavage, 68
Stacey, Judith, 167
stage theory of procreative rights, 17
Standard North American Family, 39
state laws, 135–164, 169–170; in
California (*see* California); compared
to actual practice, 142; on egg donation,
3, 140–142, 144; on embryo donation, 3,
136, 140–155; on gestational
surrogacy, 3, 140–143, 144, 151–161; in
Illinois, 52, 55; increase in number of,
141–142, 141f; on laboratory errors,
109–110; on legitimacy of donor-
conceived children, 52, 135; in
Louisiana, 143–164 (*see also* Louisiana);
in Maine, 109; in New York, 52,
110–117, 136; patchwork of, 143; research
sources on, 26; restricting IVF, 55; on
sperm donation and paternity, 3, 15,
52, 135, 139–140, 140f; on traditional
surrogacy, 142, 144, 152; and Uniform
Parentage Act (*see* Uniform
Parentage Act); variations in, 143; in
Vermont, 109–110
Stepita, C. Travers, 60
stepmothers, 31, 32
Steptoe, Patrick, 2
Stern, Betsy and William, 179–180n3
stigma and differentness, 101
stratified reproduction, 41, 169
Strauss, Anselm, 18–19
Strnad v. Strnad (1948), 52
Stumpf, Andrea, 16
surrogacy: contractual agreements in,
114–115, 144, 156, 160–161, 179–180n3,
181n11; embryo donation in, 4, 178n2;
gestational (*see* gestational surrogacy);
in hierarchy of collaborative reproduction techniques, 87, 88–89; as moral
project, 33, 35; patient literature on,
24, 82, 87–89, 93–96, 100; single men
using, 35, 176n2; as social problem,
33–34; traditional (*see* traditional
surrogacy); transracial, 126, 179n5

sweat, and kinship claims in surrogacy, 34, 84
switched at birth, embryo mix-up cases viewed as, 117, 133

Teman, Elly, 34, 94, 95, 102
tender years doctrine, 38
Thompson, Charis, 34, 75, 84, 94, 154
"throuple," birth certificate information for, 168–169, 181n1
Tipton, Sean, 116
"too fertile" story, 40
traditional surrogacy: Baby M case on, 142, 144, 179–180n3; birth family and intended parents in, 35; embryo donation in, 178n2; in hierarchy of collaborative reproduction techniques, 88–89; insecurity about maternity in, 34; patient literature on, 88–89; procedure in, 4; state laws on, 142, 144, 152
twin pregnancy: bonding of infants in, 114, 116, 178n2; in embryo mix-up case, 107, 110–117, 125–129

uncertain maternity, 6, 13, 27, 165, 166; compared to uncertain paternity, 6; in embryo mix-up cases, 25, 26, 104–134; historical examples of, 175n3; and postmodern family, 27, 166
uncertain paternity, 6, 13–14, 59
Uniform Law Commission, 109, 135–136, 142, 179n1
Uniform Parentage Act, 132, 135–136, 139, 142; in Alabama, 143; in

California, 122; on laboratory errors, 109; on parent-child relations, 20, 121; by state, 137t–138t
Uniform Status of Children of Assisted Conception Act, 135–136
unintended parents, 131–134. *See also* intent concept
University of California, misuse of cryopreserved embryos in, 70
Utah, 142
uterine lavage in in vivo fertilization, 68–69

Vergara, Sofia, 169
Vermont, 109–110
visitation rights in embryo mix-up cases, 111, 114, 116, 120, 124, 126

Walters, LeRoy, 65
Washington (state), 142
Washington, D.C., 140
Watson, James, 53, 177n7
Weick, Karl, 7, 107
Weisman, Abner I., 61, 62
Weissman, Anna, 40
West, Candace, 36
Weston, Kath, 167–168
Whitehead, MaryBeth, 179–180n3
womanhood and motherhood, 30–31
Womanly Art of Breastfeeding, The, 29

Ziff, Elizabeth, 34
Zimmerman, Don, 36

About the Author

KATHERINE M. JOHNSON is an associate professor of sociology and the director of the Gender and Sexuality Studies Program at Tulane University. Her research focuses on the sociology of reproduction and explores themes such as stratified reproduction, postmodern family building, motherhood, and medical and technological interventions in reproduction. Through this work, she has examined a range of reproductive topics, including infertility, collaborative reproduction, abortion, childbirth, and breast-feeding. More recently she started working on issues of campus sexual violence and the transformative possibilities of feminist pedagogy to create healthier and safer campus cultures. Her work has appeared in both academic and practitioner-oriented journals.

Available titles in the Families in Focus series:

Katie L. Acosta, *Amigas y Amantes: Sexually Nonconforming Latinas Negotiate Family*

Riché J. Daniel Barnes, *Raising the Race: Black Career Women Redefine Marriage, Motherhood, and Community*

Ann V. Bell, *Misconception: Social Class and Infertility in America*

Amy Brainer, *Queer Kinship and Family Change in Taiwan*

Mignon Duffy, Amy Armenia, and Clare L. Stacey, eds., *Caring on the Clock: The Complexities and Contradictions of Paid Care Work*

Estye Fenton, *The End of International Adoption? An Unraveling Reproductive Market and the Politics of Healthy Babies*

Anita Ilta Garey and Karen V. Hansen, eds., *At the Heart of Work and Family: Engaging the Ideas of Arlie Hochschild*

Heather Jacobson, *Labor of Love: Gestational Surrogacy and the Work of Making Babies*

Katherine M. Johnson, *Undoing Motherhood: Collaborative Reproduction and the Deinstitutionalization of U.S. Maternity*

Katrina Kimport, *No Real Choice: How Culture and Politics Matter for Reproductive Autonomy*

Katrina Kimport, *Queering Marriage: Challenging Family Formation in the United States*

Mary Ann Mason, Nicholas H. Wolfinger, and Marc Goulden, *Do Babies Matter? Gender and Family in the Ivory Tower*

Jamie L. Mullaney and Janet Hinson Shope, *Paid to Party: Working Time and Emotion in Direct Home Sales*

Margaret K. Nelson, *Like Family: Narratives of Fictive Kinship*

Markella B. Rutherford, *Adult Supervision Required: Private Freedom and Public Constraints for Parents and Children*

Barbara Wells, *Daughters and Granddaughters of Farmworkers: Emerging from the Long Shadow of Farm Labor*